# Who Knew?

*A Continuation of*
*You Never Know: A Memoir*

Romy Shiller, PhD

Order this book online at www.trafford.com or email orders@trafford.com
Most Trafford titles are also available at major online book retailers.

Printed in Victoria, BC, Canada.

ISBN: 978-1-4269-2654-9 (sc)
ISBN: 978-1-4269-2764-5 (dj)
ISBN: 978-1-4269-2657-0 (e)

Library of Congress Control Number:  2010903063

*Our mission is to efficiently provide the world's finest, most comprehensive book publishing service, enabling every author to experience success. To find out how to publish your book, your way, and have it available worldwide, visit us online at www.trafford.com*

Trafford rev. 5/18//2010

Trafford
PUBLISHING®  www.trafford.com
North America & international toll-free: 1 888 232 4444
(USA & Canada) phone: 250 383 6864 ♦ fax: 812 355 4082

*For Eli and Tomek*

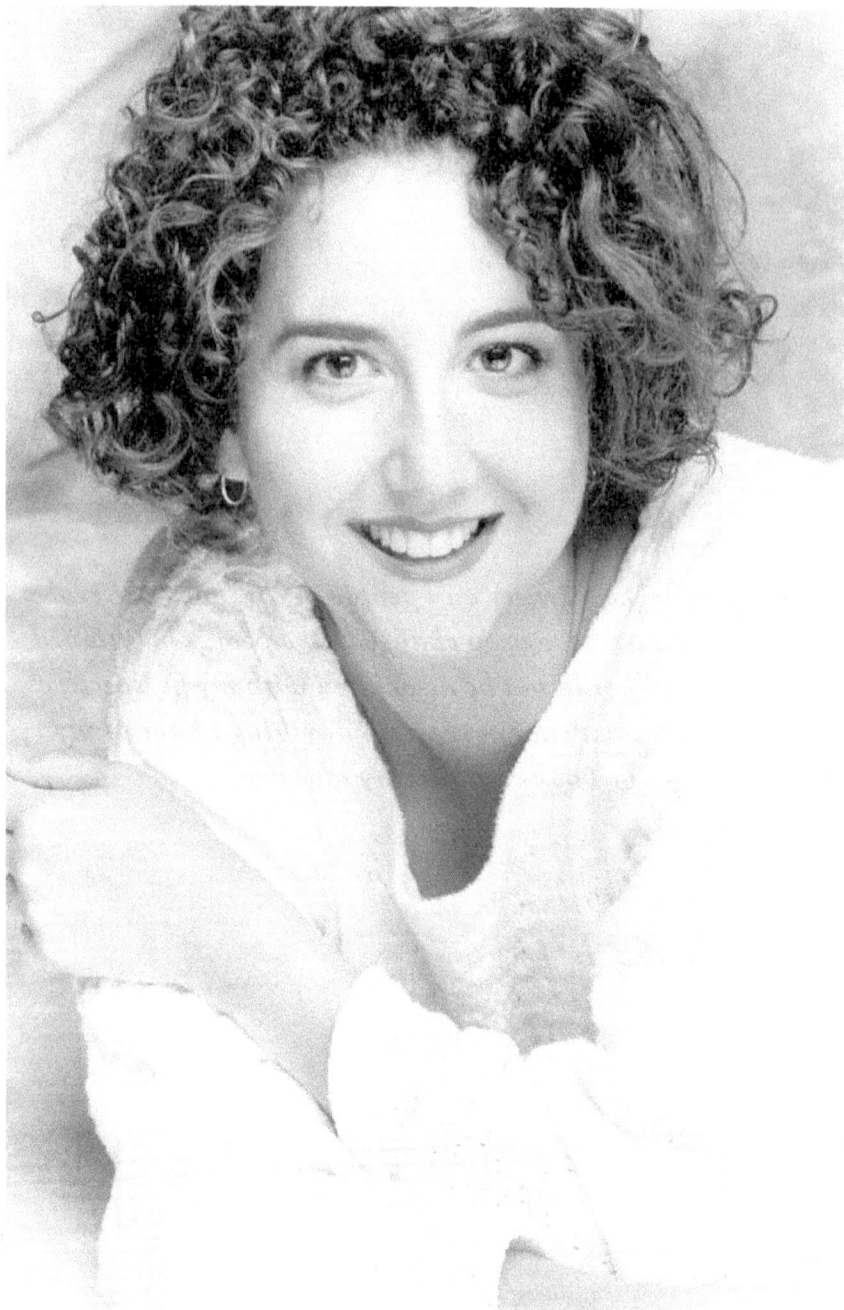

Romy Shiller, PhD

# Contents

———•◆•———

Introduction: Blah, Blah                                    ix

Chapter 1:    La, La                                         1

Chapter 2:    Stop and Smell the Roses                       9

Chapter 3:    Walking in Water                              15

Chapter 4:    Really                                        19

Chapter 5:    Yup                                           25

Chapter 6:    Face It                                       29

Chapter 7:    Suspended Animation                           35

Chapter 8:    Weight and See                                39

Chapter 9:    Much Ado about Nothing                        43

Chapter 10:   Vive la Difference                            51

Chapter 11:   Like a Prayer                                 57

Chapter 12:   Old School                                    61

Chapter 13:   Kind Of                                       67

Chapter 14:   Holy Cow!                                     77

Chapter 15:   Oh, Baby                                      81

Chapter 16:   Balancing Act                                 85

Chapter 17:   Worthy Estimation                             89

Chapter 18:   Letting Go                                    95

Bibliography                                                99

Parts of Chapter 13 can be found in my articles
"Double Standard?" and "Crush and Some Dualities."

# Introduction

—•—

## *Blah, Blah*

IF YOU ASK ME WHAT I CAME TO DO IN THIS WORLD, I, AN
ARTIST, WILL ANSWER YOU: I AM HERE TO LIVE OUT LOUD.
—Emile Zola

I DID NOT anticipate that my book *You Never Know: A Memoir*
would ever affect people, especially those who did not know
me. The main responses have been "We want more" and "What
next?" So this is less of a sequel, because of my ongoing recovery,
and more of a continuation. My first brain surgery was on August
13, 2003, and my five-month coma began a few days later.

I still continue to write books using one severely bent finger,
but it is much quicker now. Writing has become a kind of
addiction and enables a free voice. Because of my voice and
speech impediment called dysarthria, this constitutes a huge
bonus. I can express myself as I want to. The thoughts in my
mind sound so clear to me that it is a relief to get them out.
Writing is seamless, and there is no obstacle to sounding like I
used to. People who knew me before the coma said that when
they read *You Never Know*, they heard me like in a letter. My
voice has become my writing. Who knew?

When I think, sing, or write, I hear the old me. Of course,
this is inside my mind, but it is kind of bizarre. The fact that

what others hear does not match what I hear in my mind is not only discrepant but a comment on the nature of reality. This is far from fun, but I get it. My voice has become an example of what I believe. My interpretation of it regards it this way. For someone else, it would mean something else.

I actually sing in my mind much differently than I used to. A song was playing on the radio, and in my mind I belted it, which I could never do before. My voice used to be operatic, and the very high notes were sung that way in my mind. I find this cool. It might sound like I am rationalizing or coping with my new situation, but I hardly miss singing.

This book is more about the integration of my new reality than about a separation of before and after. This integration is often complicated because I have gone through the process and others have not. My new perspective is often contrary and collides with expectation.

When I write, there are many pop-culture references because that is my area of expertise. Watching films and television shows is research. I really do not articulate whether I think they are good or bad, only appropriate or inappropriate. This book is not a pop-culture critique.

People often want to know where I find inspiration. Nature is my thing, so I find inspiration in flowers, trees, lakes, and clouds, to mention a few. My perspective on the links between the environment and our economy sound like an advertising or political party campaign. My parents will jokingly pretend to hold a microphone in front of me and ask if they can quote me. Linda Hogan said, "There is a way that nature speaks, that land speaks. Most of the time we are simply not patient enough, quiet enough, to pay attention to the story."

I used to live in the sprawling city of Toronto, but quite frequently I would go to the country and take long walks through a wooded area with a trail. Sunshine would peek out from the green leaves on the big trees beside me. Twigs would crunch under my feet. The air was fresh and entirely different from the smog of the metropolis. Heaven.

Dualities—so many. Thank goodness I can hold up many things at the same time. If I couldn't, I think my attitude and life would feel tragic. I tend to hybridize a lot in my life. There are seemingly discrepant attitudes around me, but the good stuff stays with me and I chalk up the rest to lessons. It is really tough to do this.

Even though I have substantial issues with my parents, I am very fortunate to have them. I am extremely supported and always encouraged to think, write, move my body, and use my voice. I am not in an institution. They are very present in my life and take me on vacations, to museums, to films, to the theatre, shopping, etc. I have a great attitude because I can afford to have one. This does not escape me, nor do I ever take my good life for granted. Things could be much worse. I am often reminded of this when I see a disabled person panhandling on the street. Sure, my disabilities make life difficult, but life is hard. For example, when I am lucky enough to travel, there is an extra complexity. If I fly in an airplane, a special wheelchair, provided by the airline, is used to bring me to my seat. This makes me feel like a freak. It is required that I cross my arms to my chest so they do not get bumped along the way. Crossing my arms in general is very problematic. My left arm barely rises, so I need the right one to keep it in place. I am still on a plane, though. The glass is half full.

Image (the way we regard how we look) is seriously problematic here. The way I used to look versus the way I look now is not a matter of "before" and "after" in my mind; rather, it is a consequence and a result. We tend to look at most things as this or that, but I prefer blending realities and weaving the idea of identity. I am exploring where I am in my life now, and that includes image for me.

There have been several physical changes, but I think most of my changes have happened as a result of modifications in awareness. To me, clarity of mind is occurring. The physical changes continue to be very slow. Patience. Someone mentioned that it had been five years at the time since my brain surgeries and five-month coma, but because not much in my life makes me feel like a duration of time has passed, I am unfazed by this. I do mention in this book that only now am I doing certain things, but length of time is not shocking to me. I will always have dysarthria, my voice and speech impediment; I speak and sound completely differently now. I used to sing professionally. I can still communicate with my voice, though; I do not need a computer-generated voice like Stephen Hawking or hand gestures like the deaf use.

I am still in a wheelchair. My disabilities are many. I still have poor vision, so reading is slow and requires a machine for magnification. I still cannot write by hand, and the left side of my face barely moves. The word *paralysis* has been used. The entire left side of my body is different than the right. It is a great deal weaker. Using my left arm and hand is nearly impossible without assistance. I still have not sucked on a mint or candy or chewed gum. I had a lollipop the other day and thought, "How brilliant—a candy you can hold outside of your mouth!" I do not eat some foods, like popcorn, for fear of choking. I cannot swim, bringing back memories of being on a swim team. I go in a swimming pool now for physiotherapy, and I float with an inflatable device around my neck for protection. I cannot whistle. Puckering my lips—what is that? I cannot clap. There are many times after a show that I want to. The limitations of my body are extensive. I continue to feel very strong mentally, maybe even stronger than before. My body does seem to contradict strength. Physicality ... the issue of control is still compelling. I have no control over my physical restrictions, yet I feel very much in control of myself. Even though I continue to work hard with a physiotherapist almost every day of the week, these remain.

The thing is that you never know when you are going to become disabled. In the film *The Curious Case of Benjamin Button*,[1] several characters say, "You never know what's coming for you." So true. Someone sent me a video of a person safely crossing the street at a crosswalk and being struck by an out-of-control car.

Additionally, as the population ages and as life is prolonged, we should consider various repercussions. I like this quote by Charles Theodore "Chili" Davis: "Growing old is mandatory; growing up is optional." Arthritis could lead to cramped, compromised hands. Poor circulation might make it difficult to walk up stairs. A walker might be used to aid in walking. Vision gets weak. Memory could suffer. Strength is diminished. We need to think about disability now. Some things are up to chance, and some are inevitable.

The right to access for all is primary. There are places I cannot go because there are stairs and no ramp. Public transportation (will be accessible in 2029—I hope I am alive) is often inaccessible. Who is this public? I have considered moving to a different province just so that I can get around.

Sure, life can be daunting and, at times, sad. For me, perspective is everything.

---

1    2008 David Fincher dir. Plot summary: "Tells the story of Benjamin Button, a man who starts aging backwards with bizarre consequences." <http://www.imdb.com/title/tt0421715/>

# Chapter 1

―――・――

## *La, La*

A BIRD DOESN'T SING BECAUSE IT HAS AN
ANSWER; IT SINGS BECAUSE IT HAS A SONG.
—Maya Angelou

APRIL 27, 2008 — It was years since the first brain surgery (August 13, 2003) and coma, and I sang my first song. Of course, only I knew I was singing "Think of Me" by Andrew Lloyd Webber because I still have a voice and speech impediment called dysarthria. I used to practice this song at the Royal Conservatory of Music in Toronto. I was also asked to sing a song from the musical *Phantom of the Opera,* which this song is from, as a guest star with Bitch Diva (Michael Fitzgerald) at Pimblette's in Toronto. So what precipitated my singing? Well, it was Andrew Lloyd Webber night on *American Idol* (2008), which I had watched, and a young female singing prodigy (Nikki Yanofsky) sang the National Anthem at a hockey game that was playing on the television at the restaurant where I was eating. This really agitated me. I sang in the shower the next day. Later on, I sang "Think of Me" from *Phantom* for my parents and asked them to identify it. My father got it, but he said it took a lot of skill. I know I sound awful now, so I have to reconfigure the experience of singing as something I am doing for myself.

I have known for a long time that singing for me was personal, but it took a while to absorb, to not give a hoot who heard me. Billie Holiday said, "I hate straight singing. I have to change a tune to my own way of doing it. That's all I know." I guess that I am singing my own way now.

As I said in *You Never Know: A Memoir,* it was horrible for me to sing in front of my nephew, Eli. Now I sing "Happy Birthday." It still sounds awful, but at least I try, eh? I started to practice "Think of Me" in voice therapy in addition to other songs.

Initially, I was concerned that my speech/voice pathologist would have difficulty understanding me, but she thinks it is an amazing exercise and good for my vocal chords. Who can argue with that? I do not miss singing now, but it s as automatic to me as breathing. I often hear others sing who are not as good as I was but are much better than I am now. I often wonder at the comparison and irony of the situation. If I dwelt on how unfair it was, I would be doomed to bitterness. As it stands, I love it when other people sing around me. I only hope they remember that I used to sing professionally. I do not want them to stop at all; I think it is more about validation.

I watched the film *The Diving Bell and the Butterfly.*[2] I used to consider the commonalities between the main character (the book's author) and me a lot before I saw the film. He wrote his book with one eye that blinked letters, and I write my books with one severely bent finger. We both had brain trauma that landed us in the hospital and changed our lives. The gorgeous Jean-Dominique Bauby (aka Jean-Do Bauby), the former editor of French *Elle* magazine, had Locked-In Syndrome, had one eye

---

2    Scaphandre et le papillon, *2007,* Julian Schnabel. Plot summary: "The true story of *Elle* editor Jean-Dominique Bauby who suffers a stroke and has to live with an almost totally paralyzed body; only his left eye isn't paralyzed." <http://www.imdb.com/title/tt0401383/> Accessed October 22, 2009.

sown shut, and had a twisted face. He was essentially paralyzed from head to foot: "On December 8, 1995, at the age of forty-three, Bauby suffered a massive stroke. When he woke up twenty days later, he found he was entirely speechless; he could only blink his left eyelid. This rare condition is called Locked-in Syndrome, a condition wherein the mental faculties are intact but the entire body is paralyzed."[3] In the film, which may or may not be an accurate portrayal, he is very bitter and there is a marked before and after quality. I am far from bitter and regard my body now as an evolution or a progression.

The pictures I have of "before" are still me; they are not an avatar. An article titled "Avatars for the Wheelchair-Bound: The Value of Inclusion in Digital Spaces" (Theory and Research in HCI) explains what avatars are: "Avatars are the representation of the user within digital spaces, and can range from flat, non-animated pictures to pseudo-3D models that explore virtual worlds."

My history is mine. I looked at older photos for a television broadcast and came to this realization. I had to majorly revise what image meant for me. It is an ongoing process and is definitely one of my challenges. I regard my situation as an opportunity to reconstruct my relationship to beauty in practical terms. My ideas are made concrete. So for the time being, I shall stop the false comparisons. I am not only my physicality.

Some children were watching a CD–ROM I gave to a physical therapist that was like a mini-documentary. It had stuff I did before on it—some acting and singing—and me now. For the children, there was a clear demarcation, and some wondered aloud who the "girl before" was. When they discovered it was

---

3   <http://en.wikipedia.org/wiki/Jean-Dominique_Bauby> Accessed October 22, 2009.

me, they were incredulous and wondered if I would return to how I was. I know I have gone through a long process regarding my current physicality, which most people have not gone through at all. For me to see a continuity now rather than a clear marker of separation is substantial. The children's frank honesty is probably reflective of what adults think as well. I remember a cameraperson who was looking at an old photo of me with my grandparents that I have on my wall. He wondered who that person (me) was. A new attendant was also looking at pictures and assumed I was my mother.

Tamara (speech/voice pathologist) says that there are many ways a person can look different. I wear glasses now, my hair is longer or shorter, I am older, etc. Still … Look, there definitely is a before and after quality to me, and I think I would be delusional not to see that. It is difficult for me to be on the opposite end of the spectrum from where I was image-wise, but I can do nothing about it. Interesting lesson, though—I certainly do not want to misrepresent my looks, but I am getting conflicting feedback. Some people acknowledge a shift, while others say that I am not so altered.

I am now a different version of the old me. To move on, it is necessary to accept the present changes. Of course, I would like to have my old voice and looks, but I do not. I can still communicate—differently. Opting out of image ideology is so hard for me, but really I have no choice. I have agreed to do a documentary, and maybe showing people that it's possible to get past challenges will help. Going on camera looking and sounding like this is very hard, but it is worth it if I can reach people. In the *Wizard of Oz* (1939, Victor Fleming), a curtain is removed to reveal what the actual wizard looks like. The camera is lifting my curtain.

I do enjoy it when people see what I have done, but I keep thinking that my writing right now is equally, and maybe more so, incredible. My physicality is diminished, but in other respects I am achieving quite a bit.

That people regard their working physicality as "better" is kind of odd to me. My parents were at a party, and some people compared me to their son, who has major mental problems. There is no comparison. I understand that people who need to overcome challenges become a sudden comparison. We all have challenges, though. I might need assistance to do certain things and my physicality has changed, but really. I got a letter from someone who said he wished he had half of the brain I have. While I feel humbled by his suggestion, there is validation. No matter that I had brain trauma—I am more than capable.

Some people wonder if I am sad or depressed or feel a sense of longing when I see old videos of myself. Honestly, I am fine. I used to have major issues about the way I look, but there is a sense of pride in people seeing what I have done. Not half as many persons would have been privy to the old me without this exposure. Even if my lessons are that I was beautiful and talented, which I did not see, I feel privileged for having the awareness.

My positive attitude continues to surprise most everyone—including me. There is so much I could be broken about. I was so upset about not getting closure on one of my brain surgeries and my coma that I was sinking into a depression. I could have stayed in that feeling, and this might sound crass, but I chose not to. I honoured my feelings—they have not suddenly disappeared—but I decided to focus on other things. The hell of sadness was something I did not want to add to everything else. Sadness is not a choice—one cannot turn it on or off at will—but for me there was a limit. If I focus on the negative, I could bury myself in a hole. I could do drugs, avoid people, and not write books. Hide.

Since appearing on TV for national broadcasts, I have begun to take pictures. (My speech/voice pathologist, Tamara, thinks appearing on TV, doing an interview, is remarkable considering I would not use the phone with her two years ago.) I might have had substantial concerns with the way I looked or sounded on TV, but it was more important to me to reach out to people. Pictures now are less about how I look and much more about creating memories.

I do not have one picture with my nephew Eli as a baby because I was exceedingly self-conscious about my appearance. I have a new nephew, Tomek, and will make a concerted effort to include myself in photos. As the old saying goes, "A picture is worth a thousand words."

My very first photo with Eli and Tomek was taken on June 29, 2008. It was very calculated, like when I first squeezed my mother's hand and spoke after the coma; I thought a lot about it before I did it. The reality of my appearance might be shocking to some who knew me as I looked before, but I cannot control others' reactions.

I took a picture with Jeff and Bambie (friends of my parents) and my parents at their wedding anniversary dinner. I was resistant, but I am glad I did it. In addition to creating a fond memory, it was the best picture I have taken. The symmetry in my face is very encouraging. In the past, passport and medical pictures were quite wonky.

In an article I wrote called "Double Standard?" I said,

Most pictures we choose to represent ourselves are inaccurate, right? Most of us cannot stand our driver's license or passport pictures. May as well be a movie-star or look like the old me. Drag-identity is liberating. As I will often explain, to me "drag" is not "cross-dressing." "Drag" is about layers of difference. I find "otherness" preferable to sameness. If my disabilities put me on the fringe—great. If the way I think belies convention, so be it. I am glad that I have a PhD but I do not fit or follow a conventional model of that at all. My "difference" permeates many aspects of my being. The ways in which I present identities now are not false, they are drag.

Identity and image are interchangeable.

# Chapter 2

———— • ————

## *Stop and Smell the Roses*

There is a point where in the mystery of
existence contradictions meet; where
movement is not all movement and stillness
is not all stillness; where the idea and the
form, the within and the without, are united;
where infinite becomes finite, yet not.

—Rabindranath Tagore

I have always thought that nature was magnificent, but recently I saw ducks in a pond and acted like I was six years old at a great birthday party. Warm wind was rustling leaves on a tree—I inhaled. A jazz band was playing in a park—I closed my eyes. It seems like the smallest things take on a new significance now. People find it strange when I say I feel blessed. I remember telling a neurologist that I feel blessed, and she was shocked. I imagine some find my diminished physicality sorrowful and tragic. I had coffee with a woman who I am sure feels I should be miserable and unproductive. Sorry to disappoint, but I feel the opposite. While I know she does not want me to be unhappy, it would be expected. In addition to many things, I feel blessed to be here. Ducks, wind, and music feel magical to me. I do not take my existence for granted, nor do I feel small things are insignificant. In lots of ways, that which was beautiful to me is now heightened. I am unafraid of death, but life can be very good. Even though I am utterly convinced I will be fine after life and that does not take away from this reality.

I went to a small rose garden the other day. The colours were varied and quite fantastic. I inhaled. Imagine my surprise when I discovered there was no scent. So I simply stared at them. Even though the eye I see out of bounces up and down like it is on a trampoline, they were magnificent to me. I have a thing for flowers.

One does not face a life-threatening situation and not change a bit. There are certain qualities about my personality that are in the foreground now. Aging might also be a huge factor. I am much mellower, less stressed, nicer, and more productive. Certain qualities have been challenging, like patience and slowing down. It is kind of ironic and somewhat discrepant that my mind is very quick but physically I must be slow to accomplish various simple tasks, like picking up or putting down a cup so that I do not inadvertently spill the liquid inside because my hand shakes. If I think about it, I have to bring "being in the moment" to a very precise level.

I do not believe in a metaphorical "inside" of the body. I will just say that I feel as though I am co-existing with an image that feels anomalous. The outside world might perceive me in a very wrong way.

I do not want to give the impression that my life is a bed of roses. If it seems that way, I do not let it get thorny. Many things bother me, but I have discovered that my discomfort zone encompasses a very high threshold. I can bear a lot. I once had cats that completely destroyed my furniture with their claws. I did not get angry. I figured cats will be cats. I have always been this way.

I went out with a bunch of people and thought, "Holy cow, I must be strong." Certainly this thought was not precipitated by anything they did; it is just that I truly believe that most people who know me very well have a big problem with me. I often wonder: if Stephen Hawking looked different or if he spoke like most people, would his intelligence change? I do not fit into a stereotypical mold, and I am sure that for many, many people I know, it would be comforting if I did. I am not invited to several things. This is hurtful and insulting, but most of all it is so predictable. Do people imagine that if I thought I would be burdensome or if I knew the place was inaccessible I would participate? Is it better to not get an invitation or an explanation?

I am ashamed to say the following because many people do not have enough to eat, but my lack of an invitation for many group lunches or dinners deflates me. I do not think that most people I know would say, "We will not invite a disabled person." If someone's disabilities prevent access to a certain place and everybody goes there, then the disabled person is left out. This is not about blame; it is about complicity and responsibility.

There is collateral damage. I cannot access the stairs to where my nephews reside. I cannot visit them, and hence a relationship suffers. You do not have to be a genius to see the connection between disability and access here, eh?

There is a cliché involving a good-girl disabled person. I think I am very nice, but the way I think is far from a cliché. Like many people, there is disappointment, heartbreak, and challenge in my life. In a very lucky way, I see my bigger picture. I am able to negotiate the negative well.

I think that because my attitude is bizarre to most people I know, I need to explain a few things. This is not the path I would have chosen, but it is my path. Sure, it is very difficult and different than before, but there is a chance here to experience something new. I am not the kind of person who would succumb to a so-called crisis. I look for chances in life, and to me, this is a very interesting chance. Again, I would not have chosen it, but I can deal with my condition. Maybe I have the opportunity to transform how disability is perceived. That would be an honour indeed.

I was watching the film *Groundhog Day*[4] for, like, the thousandth time and realized that while I might not like my condition, my choice is to do something with it. Every day is the same thing because my physical changes are very slow. It is a long way from easy to be internally strong about this. I might not have "dark nights of the soul," but at times I want to awake. What I realized when I watched the film was that my road, my path, is to be very active without physicality. You know, I met a woman in my elevator who marvelled that she always bumps into me. "You could stay in your apartment," she said. An attendant was inspired by the fact that I write books: "You could do nothing." I try to do what I can despite my circumstances. In *Groundhog Day*, Rita says something to the effect of "It does not have to be a curse; it is how you look at it." My perspective does not regard this negatively. For me, my condition is an *opportunity* to live a new kind of life. Most people do not understand this.

> *I am not living with pain, I do not have cancer, I do not have a debilitating terminal disease. I may not have the same body as you, but I am LUCKY.*

There are two sides to a coin. If I only focused on what I cannot do, I would be doomed because there is so much stuff I cannot do now. I choose to focus on what I can do. Many able-bodied persons feel they should appreciate their status. Good,

---

4    1993, Harold Ramis dir. Plot summary: "A weatherman finds himself living the same day over and over again."<http://www.imdb.com/title/tt0107048/> Accessed October 22, 2009.

but if something does happen, it does not have to be the end of the world. People have a fear of being trapped – in this case it would be by circumstance. We are our own jail-keepers. Even a prisoner can be free in the mind.

There is so much bullshit in my life, and I know that most people can relate to this. Life can feel harsh, cruel, and unfair. At times, I want to throw in the towel for sure. I often wonder at the lack of awareness and sensitivity I encounter. Most of my anger results from other people, not my disabilities. There are people in my life with attitudes I consider very negative, hypocritical, and ultimately destructive. Maybe my expectations are too high and I have to release these because everyone is entitled to their lessons. Bummer, though. I think of what people said after the horrific events of 9-11: "We cannot let the terrorists win by being miserable or giving up." My resilience is a personal weapon. In the face of everything, I do not give up, and if I feel miserable, it does not last long. Some people do drugs or drink to deaden what they are feeling, but I am sure that does not last. And who would want to be a slave to addiction if they could avoid it?

I was going for a pedicure and thought, "*la plus ça change.*" My physicality may have changed, but I am still me. I had obviously internalized several ideas about beauty; now a pedicure is about what I like. I got a gorgeous plum shade (Siberian Nights by Opi) that I had never had before. I was wearing sandals and later admired my toes in a café. My attendant laughed.

# Chapter 3

## *Walking in Water*

I GO INTO a pool for physical therapy. There is a nostalgic quality to it because once I was on a swim team and now I cannot swim. I adore the water, although I do get scared. To me, water is calming and energizing simultaneously. It is also terrifying now. I went on a boat and insisted that I lug around a life preserver. If I cannot save myself by swimming, I would rather not depend on others for help. As a child, I was called a fish. When I used to swim under the water, I felt like I was in another world. I would often pretend I was a sea creature. Being immersed in the water felt so safe, so natural.

In my book *Again,* I said,

I loved swimming and swam from a very early age—maybe two years old. I remember learning how to dive and back-dive. A really cute life-guard taught me how to back-dive off of an Adirondack Chair at a resort I was at with my family. He had short dark hair and the smell of the wet pavement around us was intoxicating (I have an acute sense of smell). I was probably eight years old. I ended up on a swim team in my late teens. Now I cannot swim. I go into a pool for physiotherapy where I practice walking. I love the water. (pp. 66–67)

The very best thing is that I have taken steps in the water without support or assistance. Liberation. The weightless quality to the water means gravity has less of an effect. It is simply amazing to me to step without somebody helping me. The freedom we take for granted as able-bodied beings is astounding.

I continue to practice walking with my physiotherapist Franc (Francisco). We go outside of my apartment into a long, carpeted hallway. Most of my neighbors who see me cheer me on. They are used to seeing me in a wheelchair. If my left hand could grasp and if my left arm were stronger, I would use a walker. Then again, because my balance is precarious, I might still need assistance. I have so many disabilities, eh?

I was at a theatre and a disabled person in a wheelchair offered to assist me. It was evident to her that my disabilities were prominent. I am more disabled than a disabled person.

At a restaurant I frequent with my parents, a waiter brought a special request my father had asked for before, but my ordinary request was not brought and completely forgotten. I am often made to feel insignificant or dismissed.

I was asked to sit on a stool for a television show. I cannot sit on a stool because I need armrests for balance. My entire appearance on the show was put into jeopardy because of this factor. So I did not do the show, and I have yet to hear from them again. Supposedly they were fixing up things to make it more accessible. Sure. I never thought that I would be an advocate for disabled rights, but the amount of prejudice I encounter personally is huge. I do what I can, but the obstacles beyond my new physicality are dismaying.

Where I live, there is an inaccessible underground passageway to the subway and a mall. If I want to go to the mall in the winter,

I am forced to go outside in the bitter cold. Able-bodied persons are not inconvenienced at all. Very often I cannot negotiate the ice and snow in my wheelchair. I get stuck.

Maybe the amount of time that has passed since I walked as an able-bodied person does not affect me negatively or worry me because after the coma I lost my periodor one year and then it returned. So time is not a factor for me, nor is it an indication of anything. I am not in a rush. Additionally, if I never walk again on my own, my memories of having done so sustain me. The fact that I did walk does not go away. I think that, initially, realizing that I do not walk on my own felt negative, and now it is like a shifting of realities.

I now have a most extraordinary sense of smell. I heard that when people lose their sight, their other senses become heightened. I assumed it was focusing on what one has. I have been blind in one eye all of my life, and my mother believes this is why my sense of smell has always been fantastic. Even though it has always been acute, my sense of smell has actually changed. I can smell water in the wind—I know when it is going to rain. I smelled chlorine on a person who had been in a pool the day before and had showered. I can identify body wash on a person. I was in an elevator and identified the cologne that lingered there. I can smell cigarette smoke in a separate apartment from mine. Once, a person sitting next to me in a restaurant was eating a kind of fish I do not like, and I could not finish my dinner because of the smell. I watched the disturbing film *Perfume: The Story of a Murderer*[5] and thought, "I can smell like him!" Walter Hagen said, "You're only here for a short visit. Don't hurry, don't

---

5    2006, Tom Tykwer dir. Plot summary: "Jean-Baptiste Grenouille, born with a superior olfactory sense, creates the world's finest perfume." <http://www.imdb.com/title/tt0396171/ > Accessed October 22, 2009.

worry, and be sure to smell the flowers along the way." Smell and life perception go hand in hand.

I was listening to CDs that were in storage for five years (the storage unit was difficult for me to access). Like smell, certain songs or music can bring you right back to a certain moment. Certain songs made me sad and nostalgic. I thought, "Oh no, I will never be able to listen to some of my favorite music ever again!" Some relationships and experiences have changed, and my music was evocative of these. Essentially, I reclaimed what I loved about my music in the first place. Obviously, many songs are still tied to events, but they also include an entire spectrum of available alternatives.

# Chapter 4

————— • —————

## *Really*

A LOT OF what I said in *You Never Know: A Memoir* has been relegated as a strategy for coping. It is that, but it is also so much more. When you are entrenched in a belief system that values difference, marginalization, alternate realities, and transformation, my reactions make sense. I often say that I could not be any other way. My current situation might appear bleak, but I get it.

Physicality is always a challenge. We might want to be skinnier, be curvier, change genders, appear younger or older, etc. The meanings we place on bodies are many. With gyms, advertising, food, sexuality, and gender, we participate in a culture laden with body ideology. Given all of this, my refusal to "play ball" is suspect and considered weird. Wayne Dyer said, "Begin to see yourself as a soul with a body rather than a body with a soul." As you probably know, I totally agree.

This is probably my hardest issue. It is incredible to feel that I was beautiful and thin. The idea that I used to feel fat and unattractive is a significant lesson and very sad—many,

many people feel that way. Now, desiring my old physicality is fraught with irony. To acknowledge I was more than fine is kind of overwhelming. I mean, having my completely altered perspective is like waking up from a deep sleep to realize that what I thought was real was only a dream. To have lived most of my life like a sleepwalker is unreal. My new physicality is a wake-up call of major proportions. Did I really buy into the idea of image? How is it that someone like me, who questions everything, including the physical, got sucked in? Wow. The ideology of image is so strong.

In *You Never Know: A Memoir,* I problematize beauty, which changes over time, and I do say that ideology is a bugger, but I do not think that I articulated how strong the undertow is. No wonder there are eating disorders, plastic surgery procedures, liposuction, Botox, and so on. Sure, I have avoided these, but heck, I get it. An older Annie Lennox song pokes fun: "Keep young and beautiful if you want to be loved." Most of us have internalized that idea.

What is hard for me is that a limited number of people validate my perspective, so I am often sidelined. While on one hand I enjoy my difference and status as "other," I do wish others would comprehend my reactions. As I have said, if I were mentally challenged, that would be that. It is hurtful that my diminished physicality becomes a sign to many that I am mentally impaired. There is a huge gap in what people might expect and the reality of my mind.

In the animated film *Aladdin*[6], the Genie character says, "Reality ... what a concept!" That sums up my philosophy.

---

6    Clements and Musker, dirs. "*Aladdin* is a 1992 animated feature produced by Walt Disney Feature Animation, and released by Walt Disney Pictures on November 25, 1992." <http://www.imdb.com/title/tt0103639/> Accessed October 22, 2009.

I adore quantum physics. I saw Stephen Hawking give a lecture at the University of Toronto in Convocation Hall, and I am a fan of his on Facebook. My book *Again* blends quantum physics and reincarnation.

Speaking of "the real," my hospital experience was surreal. After my coma, I was on a feeding tube; I did not eat, and when I did later in rehab, my food was made mushy. I wore diapers, and when I eventually spoke, it was very difficult for others to understand me. I was brought back to a baby's reality. In retrospect, I see there are amazing lessons here about the shifting nature of reality. At the time I was in the moment, but now my memories provide me with stunning reflection. I have the incredible opportunity to make my experience mean something else. Beyond the so-called facts of a brain-tumour removal, there is philosophy and speculation.

In *You Never Know,* I also said, "Meaning and interpretation change over time. It is not that the data necessarily changes; the context does. Context can be a person or an event. Something or someone differs, and it affects the so-called facts. In many ways, the 'facts' or data are irrelevant. I think that is why our view of history alters. It is not that certain events did not take place on certain dates; it is more about how we view these events. Our perspective can alter" (p. 95). There is a chance here to create added meaning.

All of the circumstances around my brain-tumour removal have led me to further extrapolation. This is very much in keeping with who I am. In many ways I feel lucky to do this because I do not think that most people would. I really hope that by example things might change. Believe it or not, what appears to be an untenable situation can be transformed. Many of those around me are saddened by my compromised physicality. Certainly, it is strange to have this body, but it has afforded me an opportunity to reach out to people. I cannot be sad about that.

I started to write a novel (oy)—set in the 1980s, fiction—for the first time. The fact that in my imagination I can be anyone I choose, that I can be able-bodied, is reminiscent, to me, of virtual reality. When I submit older photos of myself for articles, they show what used to be my reality so I feel free, and in some ways I can be the old me. I was listening to older music, and over time the musicians' lives changed. Some are no longer alive. They are pinpointed in time, at a certain time—a document of "self."

Duets like Natalie Cole's with her now-deceased father, Nat King Cole, are a testament to the power of altering reality.

I am into life lessons, and boy oh boy am I getting my fair share of them. My lessons are complex and hard. I am very willing to "learn," but sometimes it bites. It would be nice if everything were neat, pretty, and organized. Often it is not. Life can be messy, ugly, and frenetic.

Because of my disabilities, I get to bypass some long lines and certain items are reimbursed or free. My parents call me a V.I.P. and often share my considerations. All are legitimate, and they are entitled to these benefits. I call myself a good excuse.

I know my new reality is hard for people who knew me "before" to accept. People often seemed stunned into silence. I do not believe in a "before" and "after," but many people do. What I may regard as a continuation now is "difference" to many. In *You Never Know*, I said, "Difference is something that most people avoid. Fitting in becomes a goal. Personally, I think difference is valuable. It's the 'same' that irks me. Variation is not the same as inconsistency. One can be incredibly multi-tonal and consistent. That's what I mean by 'layered'" (p. 20).

Most of the people I am referring to have not met me but have read *You Never Know* or articles about me. I can imagine that many are wondering what they would do in a similar situation. That I was anomalous and opposed people's expectations of me does not seem to be a consideration. I continue to avoid expectation and presumption. Most people are not like me at all and would have a very difficult experience. I can only hope that by my example more options become available for everyone.

I was watching one of the films I own, which I call a reality film, *Sliding Doors*.[7] After viewing the film again, I felt that even if I had a different outcome, who is to say the result would be better? In the film, what appears to be the best path leads to a tragedy.

Reality is so interesting to me. If I were mentally challenged, I would still be me but my understanding of the world around me would alter. Nothing would change but my perception. The world changes with our point of view. We create meaning. A person starving is starving, but how we perceive that situation can shift. Meaning changes—it is far from concrete, and I think that those seeking a "truth" will be disappointed. All we can know as a constant is change. Look at me as an example. I am far physically from where I was. My situation is dramatic and clear. There is no subtlety in my case.

I often use the example that Pluto is no longer considered a planet. In *Again* I examined the shifting nature of history. Pluto and history are as they were, but *we* have changed. We might want a linear progression of everything, but there is really more alteration than anything else. Faith Baldwin said, "Time is a dressmaker, specializing in alterations."

---

7    1998, Peter Howitt, dir. Plot summary: "Young Helen is fired from her job at a PR company, and when the sliding doors of the tube car close on her, we start to see what would have happened if she'd made the train, and if she hadn't." <http://www.imdb.com/title/tt0120148/> Accessed October 22, 20009.

There is a tendency to buy into the standard and avoid difference. I value difference and find it nearly impossible to conform. I know that I seek out others who avoid the mainstream. Mark Twain said, "Whenever you find yourself on the side of the majority, it is time to pause and reflect." While I might value the traditions inherent in my religion, I by no means manifest a traditional version of being Jewish.

My academic pursuits try to find a language to articulate new definitions of species, gender, sexuality, and being. While I recycle in daily life, I do try not to recycle ideology.

# Chapter 5

---

## *Yup*

I SAW MY laryngologist. Her area of specialization is the voice. She froze my nose and throat and then used a camera to look at my vocal chords. An acid burn had healed, and she reduced my medication. I was complaining about the procedure to my friend Maria, and she reminded me that I got good news. I lost sight of that until she reminded me. Her positive energy fills me up. We were best friends in high school, and we recently reconnected. It is like we took a leave of absence for twenty-five years and began again. I am beyond thrilled that she is back in my life.

I see my laryngologist once a year, and she noticed this time that my voice had a more even tone. I work on that once a week in speech/voice therapy with Tamara. The laryngologist made me do several exercises on camera that I do with Tamara, like humming and sliding from a very high note to a low one. This last exercise presents an obvious break in the middle. The laryngologist said most singers have it but know how to camouflage it. I have always had a break. The laryngologist does not know I used to be a singer, that I sang in bands and musicals and was filmed singing in a movie.

An attendant was humming the song "Don't Cry for Me Argentina" from the musical *Evita*. I used to sing that song for musical theatre auditions. I did not get melancholy; rather, I thanked her for reminding me that I used to sing that song. I really enjoyed hearing it again. We had a great discussion about how I used to sing Italian opera, and she commented that I must have gone very high with my voice. Yup. I was a coloratura soprano.[8]

I hold up many dualities in my life, and this is one of them. Negotiating apparent discrepancies is habit for sure.

I gave a CD that the laryngologist made to Tamara. She heard the tremour in my vocal chords and wondered that I had so much control. This is something I do naturally. I do not try to instill control. If there were no camera to record it, I would not know the tremour was there. There is no effort on my part, no discomfort or awareness at all.

Tamara and I hum to smooth out my vocal tone before I speak. It sounds low to me, but after my coma I spoke in a very high pitch, always. Humming actually really helps me when I am going to talk. Tamara says this lower tone is my optimum pitch and most understandable version. She says, "The lower tone seems to be optimum in terms of stabilizing your pitch, or tone, so that your voice sounds steadier." I have a great "ear" and will often correct my articulation, but talking high has been a habit and it is familiar to go there. When I first came out of my coma and for several years after, I used a high pitch when I spoke. Now when I am tired or not concentrating, I end up

---

8    "This type of soprano has a high range and can execute with great facility the style of singing that includes elaborate ornamentation and embellishment, including running passages and trills." <http://en.wikipedia.org/wiki/Coloratura> Accessed October 22, 2009.

going high. Once I was kind of singing along to a song on the car radio, and I hit all the high notes.

After we do vocal exercises, Tamara asks me how it was. I always think of how I used to sound, and the comparison is very bad. For a person with ataxic dysarthria—me now—it is usually fine. I get conflicted as to how to respond. Maybe my comparison is unfair and not applicable any longer so I should stop. The inevitableness of my analysis is so "before and after." Dichotomies are not my thing, so this really bugs me. I am unsure as to how to integrate my new voice reality. I suppose I will just get used to it, like looking at myself. Like most aspects of life, I cannot force this. It is kind of bizarre because speaking is itself problematic, but I do it anyway. I say that writing has become my voice.

*You Never Know: A Memoir* was written like a journalMy writing style is kind of *National Enquirer*-esque in the revelatory sense. I cannot stand it when celebrities go on about their lives, like it should matter. I hope I avoid that.

It is kind of amazing that I am heard differently through writing. I was going to say it is writing-drag—here I go. In any case, there do seem to be layers to my voice, and it is pretty spectacular to be "heard" on paper.

I really thought that through my writing, my parents would hear me as I was. My mother says that although she might have difficulty understanding me occasionally, she hears "Romy" clearly. To her, my speech impairment does not in any way cloud who I am. Any expression is understood and received.

Tamara's favorite quote is by Daniel Webster, who said, "[I]f all my possessions were taken from me with one exception, I would choose to keep the power of communication, for by it I would soon regain all the rest."

Tamara says, "I believe that communication is the key to any successful relationship. I try to stress to my clients that communication does not only include verbal expression. As long as the ideas are being conveyed in a clear manner, through any modality, communication can take place. Romy is a superb personification of the above, as she utilizes her gift of written communication as her voice to the world, in order to augment her oral communication. She chooses to use her power of communication to inspire both those who listen to her words, as well as those who read her books." Wow.

It is really too bad that I cannot lecture, give a speech, or read out loud as I used to. I used to be on the radio, doing voice-overs and reading from scripts at auditions for television shows or films. After I became conscious, I thought that even if I eventually walk, I will never sound the same. When I saw Stephen Hawking give a fabulous lecture on a computer, with a synthesized voice, in the late 1990s, it did not bother me one iota. There are ways to do things.

# Chapter 6

## *Face It*

I'VE NEVER SEEN A SMILING FACE
THAT WAS NOT BEAUTIFUL.
—Author Unknown

HELENE, A PHYSICAL therapist says I can hold a smile for longer than I used to. We work on my face together, and she mentioned that I have more control in my left cheek, which used to spasm when I tried to smile. Being able to look in a mirror without too many issues helps. Mirrors do not bother me like they used to. For many years I would avoid looking at myself. Now I realize that while I do not look like I used to, I am not bad looking. In *You Never Know: A Memoir,* I articulated our preoccupation with looking youthful, skinny, and gorgeous, so I will not repeat it. Ideology catches us all. I am far from exempt, even though I know better. I wear lipstick, perfume, and jewelry and use chi-chi body wash and lotion. I am a fashion victim, and although I am aware that none of this contributes to my recovery, I do not stop. Even though intellectually it is nonsense to me, I still do it.

I also do stretches with Helene. As a part of this process, I do leg lifts. Once when I was lifting my right leg and pointed my toes, Helene called me a ballerina. When I was a young girl, I took ballet lessons, and I did ballet steps before my brain operation. When I was in the coma, my mother, apparently, did ballet-class "visualizations" with me. I was watching a dance film on DVD[9] and felt that my dance training helps me now. Whenever I watch a reality dance show on television, I feel like dancing. This is far from sad or nostalgic to me. I sit up straighter, enjoy that I know the terminology, make wave-like movements with my arms ... I take pleasure in watching the freedom of movement and the agile bodies. I mean, really, even if I were able, I would not be half as good as the competitors. I was watching the television show *So You Think You Can Dance Canada* (2008), and watching Nico Archambault dance made my heart soar.

I also work on my face with Franc. He started showing me anatomical drawings from a book to illustrate the muscles we are targeting. Believe it or not, this really helps. It affirms to me that the more knowledge I have, the better. While we are doing various exercises, I visualize the muscles beneath the skin. Gross, eh?

Because I was to appear on a television show, I started to think about the position of my head, which tilts to the right side. My head also is often raised. In physiotherapy at the hospital with Linda, I was often told to keep my chin down. "Chin down, missy," she would say. My mother says that it is nearly impossible to tilt your head if you lower your head. I tried it and my head straightened out! Unfortunately, I cannot sustain this position because I have to put it so low that my sight line is affected. In the hospital, as I came out of my coma, I would stare up into space often. This was very unnatural and had nothing to do with my vision. My mother would touch my nose to remind me to bring my face and head down.

---

9    *Step Up 2: The Streets*, 2008, Dir. Jon Chu. <http://www.imdb.com/title/tt1023481/fullcredits#cast> Accessed October 22, 2009.

I grew my hair long in 2008 with the intention of eventually cutting it and giving my hair to someone who needs it. My hair has always been an issue because it is very curly and I would blow it dry straight. A camera person who was shooting a story of me and who had seen my curly hair on a few television clips wondered why I did not keep it that way. I had it blown dry straight for my appearance. When I sent my blown dry straight hair to *Locks of Love* they acknowledged my curly hair by sending me a stuffed toy called 'curly.' I guess that one cannot avoid the 'actual.' Knowing that I would chop off my long hair for a really good cause – straight or curly, did not faze me. This, I could do.

The organization *Locks of Love* says, "Most of our recipients suffer from an autoimmune disease called alopecia areata, which has no known cause or cure. Other recipients are cancer survivors, victims of trauma such as burns and rare dermatological conditions that result in permanent hair loss." What an honour for me.

At some point, I solicited thoughts from my friends and family about me and my situation, and I think it is best to share their responses in their own words. In *You Never Know*, I described how my brother Warren and I have a tradition of sending each other calendars for the New Year. At the time I had a calendar full of tractors. Now it is shoes. The shoe of the month makes me laugh hysterically. He is writing comedy for a performer now. I am so glad because, honestly, he is the funniest person. I have many funny people in my life, but Warren's sense of humour is frankly stunning. Since I was a little girl, I have said he should be a stand-up comic. He used to make the funniest home videos. I still watch them. His comical sensibility and unique take on life demonstrates how very talented he is. I asked Warren to e-mail me about our relationship to comedy. Warren wrote, "First of all,

I believe that people who have a good sense of humor are usually intuitive people in general. Show me someone with no sense of humor, and I will show you a very stiff, boring person with no insight whatsoever. I am actually amazed when I meet someone with no sense of humor, and usually feel quite sad for them."

He also said,

I think Romy and I connect on a very deep level. We always have. That's not to say we don't have our differences or haven't had times when our relationship was less than ideal. There exists a connection between us that seems to transcend basic levels of communication. I think everyone feels this with specific people in their lives. Usually you can count on one hand the number of people that fall into this category. It's a special thing, one that should not be taken for granted, although many times we do.

And so when it comes to comedy, and how Romy and I relate to comedy, and to each other, something very special seems to happen. We find very unique ways of making each other laugh, which may seem somewhat strange to the outside observer. One example is a tradition we started some years ago, prior to Romy's brain surgery, which we continue to this day, and which seems to have taken on a life of its own. It's simple, really. Every New Year Romy sends me a calendar, and I send one to her. The last calendar Romy sent me had pictures of nuns (dressed in full habits) playing a different sport each month of the year. January was volleyball, and February was badminton, I believe.... Yes, we find this funny.

I want to give one more example of how Romy and I use comedy to communicate. I don't even know if Romy remembers this. Romy was in the hospital in Toronto after her brain surgery. I would come to visit her from Los Angeles every few months. One day my mother and I were walking with Romy around the hospital grounds. Romy was in a wheelchair and completely unable to move or communicate at this point. We picked a pleasant spot and parked the wheelchair, trying to give Romy something to look at other than the blank wall in her hospital bedroom. [This was probably right after my coma.] After a few minutes, I looked over at my sister and noticed she was drooling. There was some serious drool making its way down from the corner of her mouth to her shoulder blade. Of course, there was nothing she could do about it herself. She couldn't move a muscle. I just stared at her ... drooling ... and Romy stared at me staring at the drool, and then we both just laughed! I could tell Romy was laughing because she was able to achieve the slightest of smiles. Some might view this as a cold or heartless reaction to seeing your sister completely immobile and drooling in a wheelchair, and they would completely miss the point. I wasn't laughing at my sister, and she wasn't laughing at me. We were both laughing at the absurdity of life. Romy had not spoken a word in months, yet I was able to have an entire conversation with her in that one moment, with that one laugh. This is the role comedy plays in our lives."[10]

I adore watching comedians do stand up. In my life, I laugh a lot. There is a lot of sadness around me. My laughter is real and does not negate a recognition of negativity. In my book *Again* I said, "Keep one foot firmly planted in your personal beliefs and one foot in the pool of ideology. You might get a little wet, but it is only water. Water evaporates. It is like a bridge between worlds" (p. 86).

I know it seems like I am bridging worlds. Maybe I am.

---

10    E-mail from November 6, 2008.

# Chapter 7

## *Suspended Animation*

REALITY IS MERELY AN ILLUSION,
ALBEIT A VERY PERSISTENT ONE.
—Albert Einstein

I HAVE LEARNED that there are several types of comas. I was not asleep for five months; I had sleep-wake cycles. I would open my eyes when I awoke and close them when I fell asleep. I would laugh/rasp at jokes, but I did not move or speak. I had no muscle activity in my face or body. The nurses would put me in a wheelchair so that I was not lying down all the time, with pillows to prop me up so I could avoid flopping over. All I remember are vivid dreams. I had no nightmares in five months. This was my coma.

I am asked what I remember a lot. My reality was my dreams. Warren asked if I remembered being wheeled by him and my mother to a window to look outside. He was very surprised when I said that I do not.

I used to believe comas entailed being in a sleep state for however long. Much of my knowledge was based in film or television. My own experience, which I do not remember, belied that reflection. Because there was no sudden wake-up, it is difficult to know exactly when I came to consciousness. I remember being wheeled around my floor to look at some Christmas art. It was

January. I have no memory of December at all. So January 2004 has been a marker of when I emerged from my coma. Even though I did not speak for six weeks more and although movement was severely limited (because of the akinetic mutism), this is the time marker.

When I first started to move, I would inadvertently kick people, like doctors. Sheesh. They would pad the sides of the bed in the hospital so I wouldn't hurt myself. I remember when my neurosurgeon came to visit me and I kicked him. Oy. Before I could transfer myself (with personal assistance) into a wheelchair, I was lifted mechanically—with something like a small crane—into a wheelchair. The apparatus was called a Hoyer lift. It was like an amusement park ride. I remember flying through space. I was wheeled to do physiotherapy (which hurt awfully) to a place that resembled a gym in the hospital. There was such a nice person there, named Candy. I remember her cheerful smile more than the uncomfortable physiotherapy. When I went into a rehabilitation center later, there were two assistants who likewise affected me. One of them would play board games with me. While I will never forget him, I do not remember his name. I got him a Coldplay CD—my favorite band—as a going-away gift. Alexis, the other assistant, wore a skirt I used to have. She used to talk about England, reminding me that I had adored a visit to London. Not to generalize, but everyone I met there had the best sense of humour. When I lived in Paris, my boyfriend was British. His accent was super sexy. I got Alexis some English-brand make-up as a going-away gift.

I had my first surgery at the Toronto Western Hospital on August 13, 2003. I lapsed into a five-month coma after surgery to replace a drain placed in my head to remove excessive fluid, I ended up bleeding in my brain. Two neurosurgeons needed to do corrective emergency surgery afterward.

There are layers to my consciousness. It is not like I came out of my coma as I was. In March 2008, I began to understand that I needed to shift weight so that I could sit evenly. It might seem obvious to do this, but I did not feel any discrepancy and so did nothing to correct myself. I lean my entire body to the left side. I am afraid to fall over, and I was unaware that I was lopsided. I am also more aware now that intense pressure is not needed on things like a cup handle or remote control. When I came out of physical rehab in Toronto, in 2004, a new physiotherapist wanted me to hold eggs to teach me this. I am more aware of my physical appearance and donated a winter hat that I felt did not suit me. My mother called the purchase one that was "pre-awareness." I will also not climb the fifteen stairs to the pool with my physiotherapist because an older phobia about heights has resurfaced. I had climbed these stairs for a while. I think that there are many implications around becoming more aware, but one thing is constant—my attitude. I made my first phone call on October 29, 2008. I was incredibly proud, and the person on the other end understood me perfectly. I have substantial issues regarding the phone and my voice now. This person only knew my new voice and was so nice that there was a comfort level. A few days later, I had a dream in which I was talking to my mom, explaining that this is my voice, like it or not. I later made an actual call where I asked a total stranger for someone I was looking for. Dreams can be really helpful.

Only in May 2008 did I ask pointed questions about my brain trauma time line. I also asked my physiotherapist why my right arm and hand shake when I reach for a target, like a cup. He said it was ataxia. The shaking in my right arm and hand is completely different than the shaking in my left side, which is a violent tremour instigated by things like being helped to put on a sleeve or simply being touched. It is controlled by Botox, which is not only a cosmetic drug. For me, Botox is medical—although the doctor who gives me the injections says I will have a very young-looking arm.

Moving to live on my own in June 2007 was like throwing ice water on my face. I really feel a new alertness and a substantial awareness. Also, getting new attendants requires that I focus on details. Franc said this process is like putting on glasses for the first time. One is not aware of possible clarity until there is a difference.

People wonder what it is like to lose time. Essentially time froze for me; I was in suspended animation.

In the uber-cheesy film *Mammoth* (2006), this discussion takes place:

*Agent Powers:* [Your grandfather is] frozen; all of his vitals are normal, a kind of suspended animation.

*Jack Abernathy:* Well, *The Empire Strikes Back* was always his favorite movie! [referring to Han Solo being frozen in said film].

Think about when you are asleep—time becomes meaningless. It is only when we are conscious that we realize that time has passed. My friends and family were worried that I might have Locked-In Syndrome; they thought that maybe I could not indicate that I was aware. I have no recollection of anyone or anything. I was in my own capsule of reality, with just vivid dreams, most of which were set in nature, like forests and beaches. There was a narrow lake and a country cabin that substituted for a hospital.

One day I will live in the country. I believe in making one's dreams come true, if possible. My desktop images on various computers I have owned have been of homes set in the country. I often say that if I won the lottery, I would have an accessible home in the country. Now, I am thinking I will make that happen whether I win the lottery or not. In my last book, I talked about connecting the dots. That is what I am doing.

# Chapter 8

## *Weight and See*

WORDS HAVE WEIGHT, SOUND AND APPEARANCE;
IT IS ONLY BY CONSIDERING THESE THAT
YOU CAN WRITE A SENTENCE THAT IS GOOD
TO LOOK AT AND GOOD TO LISTEN TO.
—William Somerset Maugham

I HAD STRABISMUS surgery on my left eye in January 2008. It was inverted and needed to be corrected. The surgeon said he was able to get 70 percent of it. To many, it is straight now. To me, it is off-center but much better than having an eye stuck pointing toward my nose.

Then in December of 2008, I had eyelid surgery that reduced my constant tearing and made my face more symmetrical. I had to have a cardiogram at the hospital first. Procedures, more necessary surgery ... ugh.

I have learned to read using an electronic magnification device. I call it the reading machine. Text is made larger so I can see it, but because it also relies upon being able to use body parts like my arm to move the book, it is tiring and difficult. I do not want to use books on tape—I want to read—and anyhow many of my interests, like quantum physics, just do not appear on tape. It is so bizarre now that reading has become a major obstacle when I used to do it so freely. I have bookshelves full of books, plays, and scripts I have read.

I went back to the Montreal Association for the Blind and, to my surprise, was told my vision is improving! I might not even qualify for low-vision status. I could read smaller letters than before, and apparently my eye pressure has improved as well. I never thought I would be so thrilled not to qualify for something.

It is ironic: my vision is improving, but I see a net over everything. I was diagnosed with cataracts. The "net" prevented me from using a motorized wheelchair for a very long time. One day I will have to have an operation for the cataracts, which is risky because I have vision in only one eye. As usual in my life, there is a duality here.

I hesitate to mention this particularly because anorexia and bulimia are so prevalent, but at the time of writing this I have lost fifteen pounds.[11] I am used to carrying much less weight than I have been, so this feels right to me. If I lost twenty more pounds, I would be at the weight I was before brain surgery/coma. (In the film *Bridget Jones's Diary*, Bridget calls twenty pounds "obvious.")[12] Larissa, a most excellent friend and person said in an e-mail, "I believe that all women struggle with weight issues.... You DO KNOW, though, that you are beautiful at ANY size!!!" I would really like to believe her. It is amazing that you can know something intellectually but react in an opposite manner.

---

11   KidsHealth, a project of Nemours, says, "The most common types of eating disorder are anorexia nervosa and bulimia nervosa (usually called simply "anorexia" and "bulimia"). But other food-related disorders, like binge eating disorders, body image disorders, and food phobias, are showing up more frequently than they used to...." <http://kidshealth.org/teen/food_fitness/problems/eat_disorder> Accessed October 22, 2009.

12   2001, Dir. Sharon Maguire, plot sum. "A British woman is determined to improve herself while she looks for love in a year in which she keeps a personal diary." http://www.imdb.com/title/tt0243155/ Accessed October 22, 2009.

I simply cannot believe that I am not a two hundred-pound drug addict. I have been emotionally abandoned by so many people in my life. Sad and unfair. So hard on me. I could watch TV all day, I could do drugs, I could abuse food—instead I write articles and books. We often forget that we are blessed.

Speaking of eating, there is a noteworthy freedom in knowing you have no choice but to make a mess. I will not eat in front of "new" people. Meals when I'm with dates and new friends are limited to liquids.

While filming a short television documentary, I informed the filmmaker that I would not eat on camera. There is both liberation and constraint involved. A very small child who had been informed of my new difficulties asked how I ate. I replied, "Very carefully." I am careful not to choke. As I have said, I do not eat popcorn for this reason. I often bite my tongue such that it bleeds profusely. It seems that I am not quick enough to move it out of the way of my teeth. I often have to remember to swallow, especially when I am writing on the computer. When my mind is engaged elsewhere, other effects occur. I always drink with a straw—wine, coffee, soda, etc. I drink out of a sealed athletic cup. Good for the environment and spiffy to look at, but I miss wine and martini glasses. A mug for coffee would be nice; so would a bowl of café au lait. I need to drink water when I talk for a length of time. It is very difficult for me to have milk with my cereal because liquids and solids combined are problematic. I usually have soup in my cup. I have to make certain that foods and drinks are not too hot. When I order my latte in a coffee shop, I specify that it should be 130 degrees. My precautions necessitate a very detail-oriented existence.

Given the huge paradoxes and problems around this subject, I will continue to lose weight on my terms. Being in a wheelchair for more than five years has really slowed down my metabolism, so even if I do physiotherapy every day, I do not walk. I saw a nutritionist who validated my extremely slow metabolism and, after surveying what I eat, acknowledged that most people have many more calories than I do.

As an able-bodied person, I went to the gym a lot. I would also swim. I used to go to Hart House, which was a gym, at the University of Toronto. I used the pool there as well. Hart House had a very charming and historical quality to it, which I loved. There is absolutely a difference in my physical activity now. Additionally, my stamina sucks. I do not eat excessively at all, so the weight gain is a bummer. Even though I am aware this is the least of my concerns, there is an "oy" factor. I am now a manifestation of our anxieties.

I often address the huge issue of image. I met someone online, and I used an older picture (a big "ha" for me but problematic). The girl in the photo (me) is slim, and now I am larger. He shifted as well: I thought he was a completely different person on his blog. He used a photograph that was not him. Pictures are often confusing, but in our society we learn from an early age that men can often be "less than" but women need to be stunning if not equal to an image of the man she is with (see my article "Ogre-Drag"). I do not believe pictures are accurate depictions of "self" at all, but they can often point the way to identity. He was unaware, for example, that I am disabled. I am certain, however, that his picture did not tell many stories as well.

# Chapter 9

— ◆ —

## *Much Ado about Nothing*

THE IMAGE IS MORE THAN AN IDEA. IT IS A VORTEX OR
CLUSTER OF FUSED IDEAS AND IS ENDOWED WITH ENERGY.
—Ezra Pound

SOMEONE I HAVE not seen for about twenty years, Kathy, recognized me on the street. I was on my way in the wheelchair, accompanied by an attendant, to a coffee shop, when Kathy stopped and asked if it was me. Another old friend, Maria, who had not seen me in twenty-five years, said I looked the same as I did in high school. We were at my book launch for *You Never Know*, and my attendant made a comment about me worrying about image. I feel that I look unrecognizable now, so I was completely blown away by these instances. These people had not seen the quite recent me, so I am thinking maybe my appearance reverted to an earlier time. My energy is the same, I am me, but my physicality has altered substantially. I do believe in transformation, and some part of me must have believed I had transformed almost completely.

My attendant says that I completely misrepresent my looks in *You Never Know*. She claims that I seem in that book worse than I am.

I think the way I relate to my new physicality confuses most people because it is completely different than they expect. If I am supposed to be morose and distraught, I am not. I was laughing hard in a restaurant because of something someone said and was told I seemed happier in a wheelchair than the patrons around me. As usual, I belie convention and expectation.

I am in Montreal now. Montreal is both French- and English-speaking. While the French language has a dictatorial quality to it (language "police" exist), I adore French. I lived in a quaint apartment in the predominantly English West End in the 1980s, Notre Dame de Grace (N.D.G.). I breathed the East End, so it felt like a little retreat. My place had a little balcony, and I would stare at the garden below in the spring while sipping on a cold, sparkling gin and tonic. There was a lush, forest-like feeling to my "retreat," and I often felt that I lived in the country, not a city.

I was in Toronto for graduate school and work for fourteen years. I always thought Montreal was the best city in the world, very eclectic, so it is fortunate that I am back here now. There are sidewalk cafés where one can people-watch over a bowl of steaming café au lait. My favorite bakery is on Mount Royal Street. There I have tried the very best quiches, almond croissants, and fruit-custard pies ever. I once bought a fruit-custard pie there for my brother Doug's birthday dinner. "The borough is largely composed of the well-known Plateau neighborhood, famous for its bohemian reputation and characteristic architecture" (Wikipedia). The bagels are rolled by hand and baked in a wood-fired oven at Fairmount Bagel ... do not even get me started. I used to go to a greasy spoon on Parc Avenue (officially Avenue du Parc) for Sunday brunch, and I am certain they used those bagels. Le yum. After brunch, I would head on over to a slope on Mount Royal to listen to the tam-tams (drums). So colourful and unique. They still exist.

In the fall, I would take walks around Beaver Lake (or Lac des Castors) to see the changing colours on the trees. Fresh air on my face felt so good. In the winter, I would watch the children on toboggans. Rosy cheeks and runny noses were "de règle." If I got cold, there was a pavilion nearby and I could warm up inside.

During the summer, I would watch the fireworks (International Fireworks Competition) across the water in Old Montreal. It was way before the water area was built up, and I sat on a little grassy patch of land. A friend of mine would sand wooden-round tables for a restaurant during the day, and I would visit. That restaurant is no longer in existence and I forget its name, but I will always remember the sweet smell of the sawdust.

While studying English as my official discipline (I took courses on women in film, existentialism, communications, and drama) at McGill University, I worked at a trendy clothing boutique on Boulevard St. Laurent. The street is called "the Main" by many Montrealers. It is the city's physical division of east and west. After going night-clubbing or writing essays, I would often go to a restaurant on Boulevard St. Laurent for matzo-ball soup. I would drink beer and play pool at a bar near there, La Cabanne Lux, a "resto" north on St. Laurent, that was industrial looking, and along with my fries and mayonnaise I could read a magazine that I bought there.

In an article I wrote called "My 1980s" (www.shebytches. com), I explained part of life before graduate school:

I worked in a hip clothing boutique on St. Lawrence Boulevard a few doors down from Business. "The shops are known as much for their interiors as for fashion, and the trendsetting *Parachute* boutique on Montreal's newly stylish St. Lawrence Boulevard is a sparsely decorated, airy space with a rough concrete floor, ceiling and walls, and rusted steel shelving. The heavily textured silk, cotton and woolen clothing, much of it worn by men and women both, is displayed on sloping banks of stainless steel" (*The New York Times.* "In Montreal, Where to Find What's Au Courant"). It no longer exists.

I also love winter—I belong here. My memories of skiing and skating are kind of magical. I remember skating at Parc Lafontaine amidst light snow flurries. I felt like I was in a snow globe. While I feel there are shameful accessibility issues here, I cannot leave Montreal.

My article refers to all of this. "Beyond the very influential book *Generation X: Tales for an Accelerated Culture,* we are a 'lost' generation but there is so much pop-culture to be found that we might need to reconfigure our major presence now. Compared to the Baby-Boomers, we were kind of invisible but now they're aging. It is finally our time. I'm convinced of it."[13]

During my research, I came across these great quotes from eighties movies: In *St. Elmo's Fire* (1985) the Ally Sheedy character says, "Men ... Can't live with 'em, can't shoot 'em." From *Back to the Future* (1985), Marty says, "Doc, you built a time machine ... out of a DeLorean?" In *Bill & Ted's Excellent Adventure* (1989), Keanu Reeves's character Ted says, "Be excellent to each other and party on dudes!" or Patrick Swayze's character in *Dirty Dancing* (1987): "Nobody puts baby in the corner." From 1984 the Winston Zeddemore character in *Ghostbusters*: "Ray, if someone asks you if you are a god, you say yes!"

I also was reminded of some of my favorite TV shows from that decade. Television: *The A-Team, B.J. and the Bear, Cagney &*

---

13   The Shebytches Articles, "My 1980s." Process blog: http://rshiller.blogspot.com/ December 18, 2009.

*Lacey, Cheers, CHiPs, Designing Women, Diff'rent Strokes, Doogie Howser M.D., Family Ties, Fantasy Island, Golden Girls, Hill Street Blues, Knots Landing, L.A. Law, Married with Children, Moonlighting, Mork & Mindy, Quantum Leap, Star Trek: The Next Generation, The Cosby Show, The Facts of Life, The Incredible Hulk, The Love Boat, The Wonder Years, Three's Company,* etc. ("My 1980s").

That era, the eighties, is wondrous to me. In my article I said,

I had the very best life in the 1980s, which few people know about. I went clubbing so much, danced nearly every night, had transformative relationships, worked my ass off in trendy clothing boutiques, studied, took private singing lessons, acted/auditioned and lived in Paris, France for a bit…. To me, it was about "the grand." Everything seemed very obvious and "in your face." I think it was ironically a very real decade because what was fake wasn't hidden—there was little hypocrisy. Most everything from fashion to furniture was bigger than life; much was campy. All of this was before home computers and cell phones or texting. Rap music was just becoming popular. *American Idol* didn't exist and the trend known as grunge hadn't happened yet. Raves were a future event. We were on the brink of a cultural evolution, and all I wanted to do was dance.

It is kind of like looking through a photo album—the memories! I'm not sure but this decade feels kind of underwhelming pop-culture-wise, eh? There was a lot of great stuff for me in the 1990s but frankly it paled in contrast to the 1980s. The 70s were before my time but disco seemed great to me. I would have gladly been Warhol-esque in the 60s. The repressed 50s would have been hard for me." ("My 1980s") Although Italian fashion was kind of amazing.

Now I have three attendants—not at the same time. My mom calls them "ladies in waiting," which I love. I was watching the film *Bernard and Doris* (2007, Dir. Bob Balaban) and saw some similarities.[14]

Although I am far from as rich as Doris Duke was, certain commonalities became apparent. I get items brought to me, I do not cook my own food, and while I do not have a butler, I have attendants who dress me, bathe me, and put on my jewelry and perfume. The difference is that I do not have a choice in this matter.

My parents would have paid for my college tuition. They give complete strangers scholarships. I put myself through a BA, MA, and PhD. I had many jobs. In graduate school I was awarded several paying assistantships. At the time, I had a very bad relationship with my father, and there was no way I was going to accept money from him. For me, it was all about integrity. Now my parents help me out financially with various therapies, etc. I kind of feel that it is in lieu of tuition.

I have physiotherapy almost every day of the week. Sometimes I go in a pool where I exercise and practice walking, and I get a massage once a week for circulation—le yum. I bought a very soothing CD to play during the session. It combines New Age music with very soft native drumbeats. It is almost hypnotic. I work on strength training, face and eye control, sitting balance, walking, and stretches. I have voice/speech once a week.

My life now is about writing and recovery. I hope to learn something from all of this. Because of the major expense my disability incurs, I feel like a "poor little rich girl" most of the time. I am the beneficiary of my parents' resources. I am very

---

14   "Several biographies of Doris Duke have been published. In 1999, a four-hour made-for-television mini-series (starring Lauren Bacall as Duke and Richard Chamberlain as Lafferty) was aired with the title, *Too Rich: The Not-So-Secret Life of Doris Duke.* Her life is also the subject of the 2007 HBO film *Bernard and Doris,* starring Susan Sarandon as Duke and Ralph Fiennes as the butler Lafferty. American sportswear designer Michael Kors used Doris Duke as the inspiration for his Spring 2006 collection." <http://en.wikipedia.org/wiki/Doris_Duke>

grateful, but this is not my stuff or money. There is a huge paradox because while I avail myself of their lifestyle (for instance, I visit their home in Palm Beach), it is not my life. Like I say, this is the icing on the cake—it is not the cake. Art Buchwald said, "The best things in life aren't things."

I am dependent on many levels, and I do not think people around me realize that they have more money than I do. I have very little of my own funds, and writing is hardly a money-making endeavour.

So yes, I am extremely grateful to be financially aided and very often get physical assistance, but I was with an attendant on Thanksgiving and Christmas (even though I am Jewish, it might be nice to be surrounded by family). I wonder at true thanks and feeling blessed.

I often think of a scene in the film *Sense and Sensibility*.[15] The Kate Winslet character, Marianne, says something like, "The rent may be low, but we come by it in a hard way." It is metaphorical but, in many ways, applicable.

---

15   1995, dir. Ang Lee. Plot summary: "Rich Mr. Dashwood dies, leaving his second wife and her daughters poor by the rules of inheritance." <http://www.imdb.com/title/tt0114388/> Accessed October 22, 2009.

# Chapter 10

## *Vive la Difference*

IF I HAD TO LIVE MY LIFE AGAIN, I'D
MAKE THE SAME MISTAKES, ONLY SOONER.
—Tallulah Bankhead

PEOPLE KEEP SAYING that I am courageous. I do not feel braver than anyone else, though. I have also heard that I am strong. Okay, but really, being so requires little effort from me. Difference really does not faze me, and I am used to being an anomaly. My entire life has been about thwarting expectation. I rarely think like most people. I do not fear the unknown; I kind of love it.

My present physicality feels like an extension of older stuff. I do feel like I have transformed, but for someone who made drag the subject of her doctoral thesis, transformation is old hat. Of course, things are much harder or impossible to do now, but you know, life is not easy. Am I not going to do things because they are hard? Am I going to give in? No. I do what I have to, and believe me, there is a lot I would change if I could. This does not make me courageous. My attitude is such that I focus on what I do have. I can think and I can write. To me, this is a blessing. If I concentrated on what I cannot do, like buttoning a shirt, writing in a journal, dancing—oy. Sure, my limitations suck, but feeling sorry for myself will not alter my physicality one bit.

My positive attitude now is extraordinary to some. I visited a neurologist who said most young people who develop conditions like mine really struggle with their new reality. I am all about compassion, and I wish I could take their pain away. I truly feel badly for those who struggle with their conditions. I heard about a man who had a similar operation as mine. He used to have a very active lifestyle that included riding horses for a living. He is now in a wheelchair and cannot speak. He does not want to live.

My "new" reality is in fact old. I never bought into the meanings we have for the body. I have internalized difference as a good thing. I believe in impermanence and change. My fluctuations and shifts kind of reflect my beliefs or reality. If "normalcy" were my thing then, yes, I would have a problem. Being and looking different is not new to me. It is not like I cannot extrapolate from my past. That I do extrapolate is unique, but I do it. It is my nature. If anything, I am very lucky to be accepting of otherness. Some people are scared by that which challenges dominant ways of being, but I relish the unfamiliar and unknown. My views on religion, gender, and species, to name a few, opt out of convention. Very little is absolute to me.

I was once told that I had "balls." I know it was meant as a compliment, meaning I had strength and chutzpa. The thing is that there is no female anatomical equivalent. Most things female are considered weak and negative. Think about it: "throw like a girl." I could, but will not for the sake of so-called decency, describe how most terms associated with the vagina are bad. As a matter of fact, the area known as the vagina is rarely named. For example, on the TV medical drama *Grey's Anatomy,* the vagina was called by the Chandra Wilson character, Dr. Miranda Bailey, a "vjj."[16] I try to establish power through naming in my articles, but I know in this book that would be considered vulgar or pornographic. There is no equivalent of that which is prominent, strong, or powerful in female anatomical terms. I once wrote an article, about a television show, titled, "Why Is *Queer as Folk* Making Women Wet?"[17] Shocking!

Most of my work is about change and transformation—questioning identity. In my last book, *Again*, I explored reincarnation. Some of my articles regard how we can alter or re-envision looking. Different spectator positions often belie expectation. I validate difference, otherness, and marginalization. Now I walk the talk.

An enormous lesson for me is realizing that I cannot affect a negative response to my condition. I imagine that there is fear in "difference." People might wish that I was as I used to be; I guess I want to be accepted as I am. I might really want to change certain attitudes, but that is beyond my reach.

I do my own thing, though. For instance, in some restaurants, I used to be seated near the bathroom or kitchen. Because I truly felt subjected to an "out of sight, out of mind" mentality, I now always ask to sit near the front. I will not be party to others' phobias or prejudices. I do not like the way I look, eat, or sound, but I will not hide or be hidden. My action (sitting where I can be seen) might be small, but I believe it is significant.

In *Again* I discussed "the ugly law":

Recently, I was seated to eat near the kitchen in a restaurant. I am currently disabled and in a wheelchair. My mother said it reminded her of segregation. I will never let this happen again.

---

16 "The title of the show is inspired by the classic medical textbook *Gray's Anatomy*. The series revolves around Dr. Meredith Grey, played by Ellen Pompeo, who began the show as a surgical intern at Seattle Grace Hospital in Seattle, Washington." <http://en.wikipedia.org/wiki/Grey%27s_Anatomy> Accessed October 22, 2009.

17 FAB Magazine, Number 213, April 23, 2003, 12–17

I will insist on being seated elsewhere. An out of sight, out of mind mentality will not apply to me. That this mentality by others continues to pervade is astonishing.

Are you aware in the early to mid 1900s it was illegal to be "found ugly" on the streets of some mainstream American cities like Chicago, Illinois (Chicago Municipal Code, sec. 36034) and Omaha, Nebraska (Unsightly Beggar Ordinance Nebraska Municipal Code of 1941, sec. 25) and Columbus, Ohio (General Offense Code, sec. 2387.04)? Your punishment for being caught (in) public ranged from incarceration to fines of up to $50.00 USD for each ugly offense. Here's how the Chicago Municipal Code described and enforced The Ugly Law: *No person who is diseased, maimed, mutilated or in any way deformed so as to be an unsightly or disgusting object or improper person to be allowed in or on the public ways or other public places in this city, or shall therein or thereon expose himself to public view, under a penalty of not less than one dollar nor more than fifty dollars for each offense.*

The goal of Ugly Laws was allegedly to preserve the pretty facade of the community. The disabled, the indigent and the poor were a part of society, but nobody wanted to deal with them and fewer still wanted to actually look at them. So laws were passed to keep the deformed — especially those with Cerebral Palsy and other disfiguring diseases — inside and out of sight. (pp. 14–15)[18]

I was just thinking that beyond my precautions, my disabilities themselves lead me to being very detail-oriented. For instance, the crossword puzzle is read out loud to me. In my mind, I hold the clue, the number of letters for the word, and the letters available there. Instructing a new attendant in Montreal

---

18    David W. Boles, "Enforcing the Ugly Laws," <http://urbansemiotic.com/2007/05/01/enforcing-the-ugly-laws/> Accessed September 14, 2008.

about my routine was not hard. The details about what came after what flew.

I must have always been detail-oriented. I sometimes write several books at once. This makes most people incredulous. It is not difficult for me to hold up different subject matters. I once tried to explain to a boyfriend my thought process, saying that to me, it was like many Lucite shelves in the air. Go figure. In the film *Minority Report*,[19] the Tom Cruise character touches a Lucite board that approaches my vision.

---

19   2002, Dir. Steven Spielberg. Plot summary: "In the future, criminals are caught before the crimes they commit, but one of the officers in the special unit is accused of one such crime and sets out to prove his innocence." <http://www.imdb.com/title/tt0181689/> Accessed October 22, 2009.

# Chapter 11

---

## *Like a Prayer*

NEVER FORGET TO DREAM.

—Madonna

I AM GOING to talk about spirituality. I really enjoy my Jewish traditions, I honour my grandparents' families who were killed during the Holocaust, and I can read Hebrew. My spirituality is not based in religion, however. To me, a connection with the universe exists independent of religion. I will say that I am Jewish, but in many ways I am redefining what that means. I believe in having good energy, and to me prayer reflects that. A very good woman I know, Raemeli, continues to put me on a prayer list that circulates around the globe. The thoughts and good energy coming my way are extremely positive.

I believe that my profound curiosity about reincarnation helps me now. It is not shocking that I have a new body and voice; it is amazing to me that I am given the opportunity to be aware of the change. I really feel that I can handle transformation well. My doctoral thesis, titled "A Critical Exploration of Cross-Dressing and Drag in Gender Performance and Camp in Contemporary North American Drama and Film" explored how men and women transform through drag. Now I call what I am experiencing "disability drag" and "cyborg drag" because I have a permanent shunt in my head to drain excess fluid off my brain.

I do not perceive my body as a vehicle or something my soul travels in or is contained by. That I studied "the body" and "representation" contributes to my feeling prepared. So in addition to my spirituality, a lot keeps me going and is synchronous. My life is far from "hunky dory" and I am not always cheery, so when I hear that I am positive or like "a ray of sunshine," I hope people realize this. I was once discussing my condition, and I said I found it interesting. Someone mentioned that I was detached. I thought about this, and I really feel that my perceptions about my state are "in your face" and completely in step with who I am.

Now this is going to flip out people around me because I have never mentioned it before now. I do not know if I am still in a coma. In *You Never Know*, I say I expect to wake up in an institution. I mean it. I choose to believe this is reality, but I am open to the possibility that it might not be. One might wonder how it is possible to live with uncertainty. Look, my worldview is far from the norm anyway. My ideas of reality are strange and bizarre to most people. In *Again*, I described that quantum physics is considered weird, but I ascribe to these theories. Like "faith," much of my reality is not based in proof or facts. I do not feel confused or disassociated in any way from my surroundings. Because my life has always been spectacular and the reality of my present almost unreal, circumstances do not faze me one bit. I was watching the American television series *Life on Mars*,[20] in which essentially a cop is hit by a car in 2008 and wakes up in 1973. He often says that he thinks he is in a coma. Reality—what a concept.

I am finding it very difficult to deal with the unstable attitudes around me. In a way I am lucky because I am distracted from

---

20   Creators: Mathew Graham, Tony Jordan, Ashley Pharoah. 2008. "A present-day car accident mysteriously sends a detective back to the 1970s. An American remake of the BBC series." <http://www.imdb.com/title/tt0787490> Accessed October, 22,2009.

my disabilities, but there are better ways to be distracted. I might meditate to be more with myself. I might ask a psychologist for coping strategies. I should be a mess because of my physicality; however, unfortunately, it is dealing with negativity that is hardest for me. I often understand it, even though I believe it is most often groundless and always fruitless.

I was researching a television program on which I was scheduled to appear[21] when a segment on exorcism aired and a priest, whom I resonated with, was interviewed. In all my life as someone who seems to connect with mysterious forces, I had never felt anything like this. I felt he was so loved. I tried to contact him, and I do not think that I ever experienced a greater disappointment when he did not respond. I might believe in things that certain religious people do not, like gay marriage—love is love. When Ellen DeGeneres and Portia di Rossi got married, I was delighted for them.

Ellen told *The Advocate* (a gay magazine), in an interview conducted before Proposition 8 passed,[22] "I'm thrilled that the California Supreme Court overturned the ban on gay marriage. I can't wait to get married. We all deserve the same rights, and I believe that someday we'll look back on this and not allowing gays to marry will seem as absurd as not allowing women to vote. P.S. I'm registered at Crate & Barrel" (*Pop Sugar*).

Another advocate of gay marriage is Brad Pitt. I love what he has done in the fight for equality. "Brad Pitt gave one hundred thousand to fight the passage of Proposition 8, an amendment that would

---

21   <http://www.cbc.ca/sunday/2008/05/051108_3.html>

22   "Proposition 8 was a controversial California ballot proposition that passed in the November 4, 2008 general election and took effect on November 5, the day after the election. It changed the California Constitution to add a new section (7.5) to Article I, which reads: "'Only marriage between a man and a woman is valid or recognized in California.'" This change restricted the definition of marriage to opposite-sex couples, and eliminated same-sex couples' right to marry, thereby overriding portions of the ruling of *In re Marriage Cases* by "'carving out an exception to the preexisting scope of the privacy and due process clauses'" of the state constitution. The proposition did not affect the existing domestic partnerships registry." <http://en.wikipedia.org/wiki/California_Proposition_8_(2008)> Accessed June 16, 2009.

outlaw gay marriage in California. Brad's donation is the biggest that any A-list celebrity has donated to this date. But it comes as a shock that Ellen *DeGeneres* or Portia haven't given a penny to the cause. Rumors have it that eleven million dollars has been raised to fight Prop 8." (Associated Content)

This appeared in another publication: "Brad Pitt, ever the social activist, says he won't be marrying Angelina Jolie until the restrictions on who can marry whom are dropped" (Advocate.com). Way to go, Brangelina!

As for the priest I tried to contact, I thought our common ground was spirituality, even though I am Jewish and fairly unconventional. The result was a stunning and very unexpected lesson. That was not enough, obviously. I know that religion is a contentious issue for many people; maybe I felt exempt from this. Another priest in the piece articulated that the devil makes it feel like "he does not exist." Does the priest whom I resonated with think I am the devil? It is bizarre because I have never felt so naive and so radical simultaneously.

I saw Madonna in concert during her Sticky & Sweet Tour.[23] An article titled "The Religious Affiliation of Pop Singer, Actress Madonna" says, "Madonna was raised as a Catholic, an influence which showed up in various ways in her musical career, including in the choice to use only her first name as her stage name. (Her birth name is Madonna Louise Veronica Ciccone.) Madonna was essentially a lapsed Catholic during much of her adult musical career, until she converted to Kabbalah."[24] She is a godsend.

---

23  "The *Sticky & Sweet Tour* is the eighth concert tour by American singer-songwriter Madonna to support her eleventh studio album *Hard Candy*." <http://en.wikipedia.org/wiki/Sticky_&_Sweet_Tour> Accessed October 22, 2009.
24  <http://www.adherents.com/people/pm/Madonna.html> Webpage created 10 October 2005. Last modified 21 November 2005.

# Chapter 12

## Old School

THE WHEEL IS COME FULL CIRCLE.
—William Shakespeare

IN THE 1980s in Montreal, I went to Town of Mount Royal High School. I met some incredible friends and teachers there. Of course, there were cliques and horrendous experiences—it can be very trying to be a teenager[25]—but on the whole my experience was transformative. So many friends from my past have reentered my life. Several, like Maria and Lisa, are from high school, and I have had a PhD for years now. Maria said, "We were thirteen years old and I had just switched to a new high school, never an easy situation ... especially at that age. Romy was inviting, articulate, intelligent and held herself with a certain dignity that escapes most adolescents. I was drawn to her confidence and sense of self that shone through so vividly." I will always consider Maria family.

In many ways I have come full circle but with a new body, voice, and degree. Strange—my friends have not witnessed certain changes over the years. My looks had altered substantially, but now I kind of look like the old me. Over time a lot has happened

25 See my article, "POP goes the Teen." <http://www.shebytches.com/romyshillerjune2009.html>

to all of us, but essentially we are the same. To me, this is a fantastic lesson about time and personhood. For some, marriage, kids, school, jobs, and travel fulfill them. I like that these people knew me when my physicality was different. It is also spectacular that some things never change.

Lisa said,

When we are together it's like no time has passed. I read Romy's story in the newspaper. Instantly, I was sucked back into a time machine and became seventeen again. Romy and I co-starred in the school play (*The Miracle Worker*). I instantly e-mailed her. "Hi Romy - do you remember me?" I said. Isn't it funny that we remember someone so vividly from our past—yet somehow think that they have forgotten all about us? Romy and I started a fast and furious email dialogue and ultimately met up in Montreal. The connection was magical and we just slipped right into gossiping about high school days and catching up on our lives. We are still seventeen years old and hanging out at the front entrance of TMR High talking about whatever. In each other's eyes we look the same—I totally would have recognized (Romy) wheeling down the street. Our years of silence were totally irrelevant.... We are forever seventeen. I actually believe it is these friendships that keep me looking and feeling so young—because to be quite honest—I don't feel a day over seventeen.

Lisa has two amazing young daughters.

In a review, the author called me unconventional. I am. I know that in many paradigms, I am "other." *Normal* is my least favorite word because it ostracizes many. I rarely, if ever, use it. When my speech therapist calls my voice my "new normal," I know exactly what she means but wonder what else she could call it. My "new standard"? Maybe I will have her call it that instead.

In my twenties I worked with a woman named Nathalie in that trendy clothing store in Montreal. I adored her and admired her ambition. She became a very close friend of mine, and we both ended up living in Toronto. She said,

When I met Romy, there was an immediate familiarity; we became friends quickly and I looked up to her as someone who was living life on the fringe, unapologetic about her beliefs. She was vocal, expressive and artistic. I always thought she was courageous. My world at the time was pretty limited, even repressed. I held beliefs similar to Romy's but felt unable to express them and meeting her was like an "activation" of sorts … the beginning of an opening. She opened my eyes to issues of gender, identity, tolerance and socio-cultural change. Oh, and we danced. We danced a lot.

We recently reconnected, I am very glad to say.

I cannot even remember how Nettie and I met, but she and I became very close quickly and briefly in Toronto—she soon after moved to Vancouver. Nettie is brilliant, a gifted architect, and very generous. She also cannot remember how we met and jokingly said, "The most reasonable explanation I am sure is that we met in a past life!" We lost touch and were searching for one another on various Internet networking sites. Luckily, she found me on Facebook. On her Facebook page, she says, "You met randomly in TO - we learned, we laughed, we lived, we left." Nettie absolutely kills me. Her sense of humour is truly fabulous.

Nettie said further,

My memory of my time in Toronto is distorted. My memories of Toronto seem to span years, at least a few lifetimes. In reality I was only there one year.

This feeling can also coincidentally, be applied to my friendship with Romy Shiller.

I cannot remember how we met. It doesn't really seem important. We just were. In that one year, Romy was my constant. I feel like I have always known Romy. I may not have known actual details of Romy's life before Nettie (LBN). Those details don't seem important. Who she knew, what she did before we became friends weren't what our connection was about.

We just fit. We understood each other on a level that had nothing to do with practical everyday tasks. We were different but even our differences made sense somehow. How can I explain our connection? Words don't seem to work although I understand the necessity of finding the right words.

I've always believed that the people we meet can fall into three basic categories: a) Reason b) Season c) Lifetime.

Sometimes we connect with people for a specific *reason*. There is definitely a common element that keeps this kind of relationship active. When the common reason goes, often so does the friendship.

Sometimes we connect with people for a *season*. This is harder to explain. It's based upon connecting with someone for a short but often intense period of time.

Then there are those that we know we will know for our *lifetime*. It's not about day to day stuff. These are the people you know that no matter what, you can call at any time when you need help. These are the friends that you can lose contact with and know with certainty that when you meet again, everything will be the same. No excuses are needed for time spent away. They are always there in your heart and you are there in theirs. It's a mutual feeling that has a timeless quality and is based on a feeling of infinite trust. I am not saying you can ignore these friends. It's just that the connection is so solid that you don't need to maintain it and work for it in the same way as some of the other types of friendships. There are no conditions. Perhaps that's one of the keys. It is definitely not something you take for granted. Quite the opposite. It's something that is so cherished that you know it will never go away.

When I moved from Toronto, Romy and I kept in touch. She came to visit me and we were the same as always. Then I moved, and Romy moved and we lost each other. For years I have searched on and off for Romy.

Thank God for *Facebook* and the internet! But then, I always had faith that we'd find each other again!

I will always love Nettie unconditionally.

There were many amazing friends in Toronto. There was Daniel. I love his energy. He said,

I met Romy, and she certainly had this underground vibe but it was all sweetness and total sexiness. She had this very meta quality to her as if she was a very mature spirit who was open to anything. She instantly made me feel so comfortable probably because we had this incredible chemistry together. Within weeks we were new BFF's and connected on so many levels, most especially about past lives and also the spirit world.

I met Andi Davidson in the early 1990s. She is a musical sprite. We formed a band together in the early 1990s.

It was the year 1992 that the universe brought Romy Shiller into my life.

Romy was into "kitsch" (a term she introduced me to); her kitchen table was from the 50s and she had little postcards of pin-up girls in her washroom.

When she found out I was a singer-songwriter she asked me if I would like to collaborate and maybe do a few gigs together. We called ourselves Mystic Muse and played a few Toronto coffee houses as well as wrote a song together called "Pieces of You." I think I may still have a cassette recording of it somewhere in all my boxes of old stuff.

The other thing I really remember about Romy was her ability to read Tarot cards as well as channel divine entities. If I close my eyes I can almost see her long and narrow face framed by her curly hair, squinting her eyes as she concentrated on the messages she was to offer. It may have only been a short period of time in our lives that we shared together, but what we did share was deep, penetrating and somehow kept us connected.

When I heard about Romy's coma all these years later and then saw her clip on CBC (Canadian Broadcasting Corporation) News, I was, needless to say, shocked! How could this happen to such a vibrant and healthy individual? But it did and it does, and it is a reminder for us all to count our blessings and our fortunes. I think that Romy is an inspiration on the effects of positive thinking and believing, for determination and fulfilling our life purpose. She never gave up, she does not wallow in the sadness of her state, she continues to reach out and touch people with her sass and vibrancy. I am honored to know her!

I have been so lucky in my life to know extraordinary people. Most are courageous, smart in their own way, and very strong. We have all blended realities and inspiration. My relationships with my friends have been absolutely magical—sparkling. Each one is unique and gifted. To them all, I say, "Promise me you'll always remember: You're braver than you believe, and stronger than you seem, and smarter than you think" (Christopher Robin to Pooh, by A. A. Milne).

# Chapter 13

## *Kind Of*

I KEEP FALLING for inappropriate people. It kind of makes sense. I have always pushed the envelope, so doing this is not anomalous. Also, rejection might be easier to bear. Funny, being aware of this stuff does not prevent me from desiring inappropriate object choices.

I know that I adore it when people think outside the box. In these cases, I would force the issue and make sure that a relationship with me was very different. My disabilities are kind of subsumed by desire. Difference is manifested differently. At this point, I am living in my head as none of these have manifested into anything. That is so safe, eh? For instance, I fell for a gay man once who lived halfway around the world. Totally inaccessible, right? I am such a case. I had a dream about him. Me and dreams—oy. Anyway, in the dream he was passing me something and our hands simply touched. We looked at each other, knowing this was illicit. Hot and erotic—just hands.

A guy flirted with me the other day at a restaurant. I was absolutely stunned. He was so cute, and I thought, "He could have anyone. Why me?" Obviously, I have a problem with self-acceptance.

I was thinking, "Who would fall for a disabled feminist?" For one, there is a misperception that feminists hate men or are anti-men. We are just pro-women. My many disabilities mean I cannot rely upon image to help out. Cosmetic Botox and liposuction are meaningless to me. I cannot, like many people, wish I were younger or curvier, as if those changes would make a difference. I love that those things do not apply to me—they never did—but it might be nice to fantasize an option. I might have to reconfigure. For example, I adore male eye candy, which is as realistic as looking at *Playboy*, yet I am far from a beauty.

I have been single now for the longest period since I was sixteen. Yes, I have had to deal with loads. I do crave a relationship, though. I have major hope. My friend inspired me. She lost her husband more than a year ago and goes on dates now. She has been out of the "scene" for over twenty-five years, but she challenges herself to try. I know she will always love her husband who passed, but she is moving on. Amazing.

David Cook sings about being kissed on the neck—dreaming is good. So what do I want? Sex and a relationship. Both. With someone who rocks my world. I have so much to offer, but my physicality... I honestly believe that how I look now is problematic for many men. That sucks, eh? I enable "the gaze" for women in most of my articles. Women are sexual, play with gender roles, and inhabit various subject positions. Women are free. The big fat irony is that I feel constrained. If "come and get it" were an option, that'd be swell, but it is not.

Julia Pearlman wrote an Internet article titled "Sex When You're Disabled." In it, she said, "Being disabled doesn't mean you can't have a good sex life, but you may need to make a few adjustments to make things as enjoyable as possible" (TheSite. org). Le oy.

There is something very intimidating about having sex in a different body, and for someone extremely liberal to say that is something, I assure you. On one hand, it's an amazing opportunity to start anew, to explore my comprehension of "lessons." On the other hand, it's incredibly scary. Imagine.

An extremely bright man I know said, "Intimacy is about getting past obstacles, to various kinds of truth, communicating without obstacles or fear. One never knows whether other people mean the same things, but over time you hope to discover a consensus. Your past decade [actually half of that] has been an assault on all that, as so many of the things you used to be able to count on have been problematized or at the very least re-opened. Relationships are difficult enough when you're a shiny new twenty-year-old who can take [your] beauty and intelligence for granted."

He also said,

That interconnection you allude to in passing seems particularly rich, between human and machine, between our minds and the various extensions we now can attach. We have phones and keyboards for sending, various devices for receiving, to say nothing of the many ways our memories and senses are augmented. While on the one hand, you walk and dance slower than you used to, you have other tools that allow you to take giant strides and speak with a fantastically amplified voice, reaching many, many people. In your publishing career and its interconnections through blogs and social networking sites, you're another sort of cyborg (as are we all after a fashion).

I am currently writing a novel in which a sexy young woman makes love to her very hot boyfriend (sounds much too Harlequin). I can be any character I want, and while being virtual is amazing, there are real limitations. Ayn Rand said, "Every man builds his world in his own image. He has the power to choose, but no power to escape the necessity of choice" (Thinkexist.com).

I adore the dreamworld, but it's like the film *The Matrix* (1999), eh? The character Morpheus in the film describes what the Matrix is: "It is the world that has been pulled over your eyes to blind you from the truth." An article by Nancy Shute, "Girls With Sexy Avatars Face Greater Risks Online" (May 26, 2009), says,

Do you know what your daughter's online avatar looks like? If it's sexually provocative—more Bratz than American Girl doll—it's time for a chat. "I'm amazed at the grotesqueness of some of these avatars," says Jennie Noll, a developmental psychologist and associate professor of pediatrics at Cincinnati Children's Hospital Medical Center who asked 173 teenage girls ages 14 to 17 to make avatars, then rated their provocativeness— skimpy clothing, body piercings, exaggerated curves. Girls who created provocative avatars were more likely to get sexual come-ons online, not surprisingly, and also more apt to agree to an in-person encounter with someone they met online. Noll's study is published in the current issue of *Pediatrics*. The girls who chose provocative avatars were also more likely to be preoccupied with sex—and, Noll speculates, they might be more likely to try on the role. (usnews.com)

Okay, I won't speculate on the meanings associated with *provocativeness*. I do want kids to be careful, though I might question the ideology here. A famous Macbeth quote says, "Look like the innocent flower, but be the serpent under't" (Act 1, Scene V).

My "Bratz doll," as Shute says, is hardly "offensive." I use it on various Internet sites. I think it is kinda cute. Predators do exist, though, so watch out. "Young adolescents are the most vulnerable age group and are at high risk of being approached by online predators. They are exploring their sexuality, moving away from parental control and looking for new relationships outside the family. Under the guise of anonymity, they are more likely to take risks online without fully understanding the possible implications" (webAWARE).

I say that "identity is drag," and I'll often post my profile picture on Facebook as a glamorous Hollywood actress. My author picture is of me as I used to look.

"When you don your avatar and join thousands of other people who are trying out life in virtual worlds you are joining in a great new experiment in human contact." I was invited by a lovely gay man to participate in a site that included virtual sex. I couldn't do it. Participating would be great for my status as an academic, third-wave feminist, etc., but my preferences seem to outweigh all of that. Am I simply enacting prescribed ideology, a double standard? I am very aware of the limitations for women, and I think that I'm on the outer edge of that. So there appears to be a dichotomy. (Parts of the above can be found in my article "Double Standard?")

Wow. To be an unmarried woman over forty years of age is so suspect. I certainly could have gotten married and will, one day. I remember having an older teacher in high school who was unmarried, and I definitely prejudged her. I was not outside of ideology or expectation. It is kind of bizarre to be in a similar situation now. In my thirties I was working on a master's degree and a PhD, and I studied singing at the Royal Conservatory of Music. I had a band. There were relationships and jobs. I acted on film and a TV series and in theatre, wrote articles, studied

French, and took seminars on photography and voice work. Sorry if marriage was not a priority. I feel like it does not matter what else I did, marriage would have been viewed as a measure of success.

I know that I met a soul mate (I believe in several). We met completely by accident, and our commonalities are frankly astounding. As Brandon Boyd said, "This isn't coincidence; there's no such thing." Even for me, it is so otherworldly. He is younger than me and able-bodied. For many reasons, I let him go. My friend James would have warned me not to be a martyr. Maybe it is partly that, but it is also realistic. Hopefully, moving on will be possible.

There is such an emphasis in our culture on looks that, frankly, I imagine I will have a very difficult time. I am drawn to male eye candy, but I know better. I had a huge crush on Maroon 5 front-person Adam Levine.[26] This was absurd to me; I never have crushes on celebrities. But I found him exceedingly talented and handsome. Oy. I think that the only time I wished my new disabilities would just vanish was when I contemplated dating him. I "followed" him on Twitter[27], and he was in Europe commenting on stuff I really related to.

He has a reputation as a playboy, but "[c]ontrary to popular perception, Levine describes himself as a shut-in who quickly learned the paparazzi-fuelled spotlight was not for him after *Songs About Jane* exploded, selling more than 10 million copies and rocketing him to superstardom" (Dose.ca). Jane-shmane.

This is so cougar-esque of me—"an older woman who sexually pursues men at least eight years her junior" (Wikipedia). I was thinking of references and came up with Ashton and

26  "Since debuting in 2002, the band has sold over 10 million albums in the United States and nearly 15 million worldwide." (*Wikipedia: The Free Encyclopedia*).
27  "Twitter is a free social networking and micro-blogging service that enables its users to send and read messages known as *tweets*." (*Wikipedia: The Free Encyclopedia*)

Demi—more pop-culture. Predictable. An article online says, "So, Ashton Kutcher, 27, and Demi Moore, 43, got married with her kids and ex-husband in attendance. Hollywood ho-hum? Made in heaven? Bizarre? Insane? A giant step for women? How about 'A giant step for older women'?" (Ezine@articles).

In my book *Again,* I did say that time and space, let alone age, do not matter, and I really could look at all of this in that light. I guess that because I did not know Adam Levine, I let the dominant ideology persist. In my book *You Never Know: A Memoir,* I said, "I have always been fascinated by the nature of 'reality,' although I believe in consequences for our actions" (p. 44). I really enjoy thinking about "reality."

I went to a coffee shop I frequent and saw Adam Levine's doppelganger. I only glanced so as not to be obvious or seem perverse or something. I was leaving, and he was heading for the counter. The eye candy … no doubt some of my gay male friends would agree.

I kind of wish I looked like a supermodel, but I may have wanted that no matter what. Superficial, eh? The one area— my physicality—that has always been problematic for me is compromised. It is easier for me now to believe I have reduced chances with my crush because I'm disabled. How's that for a rationalization? In *You Never Know: A Memoir,* I said, "I have heard 'if only you were as before.' Heck yeah, but I am not; and if I stay this way, I still figure I have lots to offer. Sure I look different, but if that is the measure of my worth, that would suck. I do not buy into that. No matter how difficult my issues about body image are, I have a hard time believing that" (p. 38). I hope that my words really sink in. Peel Public Health's website says this:

*Healthy body image means feeling 'at home'
in your body—it's part of who you are....
You're so much more than a body!* Yeah.

It's nice to have a fantasy—no matter how unrealistic.

I hear Adam has dated Natalie Portman and Cameron Diaz. Beauties. This cannot be healthy for me mentally. There is what is known as the "cult of celebrity." Look at an essay called "Star Struck" by John F. Schumaker, in which he says, "A banal cult of celebrity is spreading round the globe." I do not have "celebrity worship syndrome" (Schumaker), and I am very objective about my pop-culture work. I guess my crush is run of the mill. It would be kind of relieving to relegate it as a syndrome. Oh, well.

I decided to work on my novel while I was in the realm of fiction. Even though I listened to Adam Levine's music while I wrote, I was focused. I imagine I can channel this energy into one of my characters. I like myself too much to let this get the better of me.

I can think of a million and a half reasons why I have a crush on this person. So why doesn't reason take over? I am a very smart person.

The fact that I chose a singer to gush over is not lost on me. I used to sing a lot, but now I cannot.

I listen to music a lot, like before. The difference in my voice now has not changed that. I hold up many dualities in my life, and this is one of them. Negotiating apparent discrepancies is habit for sure. I am ambivalent about my physicality, and I pick someone who apparently values the physical to have a crush on. How's that for discrepant?

Willa Cather said that "[a]ll the intelligence and talent in the world can't make a singer. The voice is a wild thing. It can't be bred in captivity. It is a sport, like the silver fox. It happens." I guess that I feel like a singer no matter what I sound like. It has always been a part of me, my past. Nothing, absolutely nothing, can take that away from me. I think that I feel that other singers would get that. Of course, I would like to sound like I did, but I feel that a part of my process is simply accepting where I am. I still have a very hard time using the phone, though. I feel that I might thwart people's expectations for sound. I also sound mentally challenged. So I have issues but no baggage. (In a form, the above can be found in my article "Crush and Some Dualities.")

At a function, I was asked to dance by an able-bodied man. When I said that I cannot, he suggested that I could sway in my wheelchair unless the experience made me uncomfortable. He also mentioned something to the effect that I should be able to partake in enjoyable activities. I already knew all of this, but to hear someone else say it was kind of incredible. He made my night.

# Chapter 14

## *Holy Cow!*

MYSTERY IS AT THE HEART OF
CREATIVITY. THAT, AND SURPRISE.
—Julia Cameron

WE OFTEN WONDER at the seemingly impossible, but you never know. I often say it's important to try what seems like the impossible—you might be surprised. People are in awe that I write books with one bent finger. This is a part of my survival technique. To me, it is a worthwhile hardship, one that I adore— writing. Certainly it is not easy, but to me it is not impossible. I suppose in life there are many things we do not try because we fear they are impossible—for instance, a new career or a hobby like skydiving, singing, dancing, painting, drawing, and so on.

Fear of the unknown seems to be a catalyst to being frozen. We have a fear of letting people down or of failure. As I said in *Again,* I once heard that the opposite of love is not hate but fear. Additionally I said,

Exploring the unfamiliar might invoke a host of emotions like fear. We obviously try to avoid fear, yet haunted houses and roller coasters are pretty popular. The unfamiliar can be thrilling and entertaining. Fear can be enticing. Scary movies make huge profits. Funny, I do not watch horror films or engage in any fearful activities, yet I am more than willing to explore the unknown. My friend Lisa said that she explores the known and I, the unknown. She says, "In school I always loved math, science and history—because it was a known." She says that I am the yin to her yang:[28] I need more yin! (*Again*, p. 120)

We owe it to ourselves to be loving, so working through fear is necessary. Obviously, we do not all need to skydive, but if that is something you have always wanted to try...

In *Again*, I said, "I once heard that the opposite of 'love' is not 'hate' but 'fear.' So let us avoid fear just in case, okay? We can take an adventure into the unknown. What we do not know does not have to intimidate us. We can explore new frontiers like the Starship *Enterprise* (*Star Trek*, 1966). I keep thinking of territories that have yet to be explored (p. 60)."

Exploring your own unknown territories is very exciting! An adventure can begin with you; you do not need to go anywhere. The journey of self-discovery is immensely rewarding. Avoiding hurting someone emotionally is a lofty goal, but one cannot always control others' emotions in reaction to one's actions. I do not think it is selfish or self-serving to be happy. There are reasonable and unreasonable actions that precipitate this. It is just plain heinous to be abusive in any way. What I am referring to is simply articulating how one feels. If a reasonable manifestation arises, it does.

Attempting something and not succeeding is not failure. Attempting can be heroic. In the film *Nim's Island*,[29] a recurring theme is to "be the hero of your own life." So what are your challenges?

---

28   Svebor Hlede, "The Meaning of Yin-Yang," <http://fly.cc.fer.hr/~shlede/ying/yang. html> Accessed September 4, 2008.

29   2008. Dirs. Flackett, Levin. Plot summary: "A young girl inhabits an isolated island with her scientist father and communicates with a reclusive author of the novel she's reading." <http://www.imdb.com/title/tt0410377/> Accessed October 22, 2009.

My philosophy is "try." I suppose if I can impart anything to others, that would be it. It feels precarious to try because of the myth of failure. It is worth a risk, even if you buy into the false ideology.

I will try to be more straight-forward. I will say it like it is—to me. The risk here is being disliked and unpopular. The ramifications are terrifying to me, honestly. Believe it or not, for someone so outspoken I am extremely quiet and fairly unprovocative. It will take a major effort to be otherwise for me. It is worth it here to honour my truth.

# Chapter 15

## *Oh, Baby*

I DO NOT even know if I can have a baby; I never got pregnant. I wanted a baby, but I always figured there would be time. My heart breaks at the thought of not having a child—my only regret. I think I would have been a spectacular mother. I was willing to be a single mother, and I even perused a sperm-donor list. Even though I was in relationships from the age of sixteen well through my thirties, I had a feeling I would have to do this on my own. It never bothered me. Sure, it would have been hard, but people do it all of the time. I even had names picked out. For a girl, 1) Gala, 2) Hero, or 3) Lux; for a boy, 1) Jackson, 2) Clayton, or 3) Clive. Oy. I remember being at work in my twenties and making lists of baby names. I asked gay friends if they would consider donating sperm. I used to peruse baby and maternity stores. Two of my close friends had abortions, and while I completely support a woman's right to choose what goes on with her body, I would never have had one. That is my choice. I always wanted a child. I take folic acid (prevents spina bifida)[30] every day—you never know. I was watching the film *Revolutionary Road*,[31] and the main character, April, dies because of an abortion she performs on herself. I am so glad that safe, medical abortions are available now.

My speech therapist will ask me questions on the phone as practice. My favorite is when she asks me about adopting a child. One day I hope I will. I attended Brooke Muller's baby shower (married to Charlie Sheen, expected twin boys). Very glam but extremely bittersweet for me.

Like I say in *You Never Know*, having children would be problematic for them and me. I still think I would have managed. My nature is to meet challenges, not avoid them. Needless to say, I would need help in raising them, but I know I could do it.

I have very adorable toddler-age nephews, Eli and Tomek. I am aligned with the dramatic, so I will simply present the facts. You may want to take this with a grain of salt—you may not. On occasion, Eli recoils when I go to hug him, and he usually shakes my hand. I would *never* force a child to be hugged, even if it is my impulse. He asked my mother, his grandmother, "Are we family?" even though he sees her heck of a lot more than me. My dad sang to him afterward "We Are Family" by Sly & the Family Stone. To me, this is all very sad and tragic. If I have learned anything from my "ordeal," it is that kids frankly say what they mean. It is often crass, but it is so honest and unguarded.

Eli and his family visited me in Florida. Warren, my brother, also came from quite a distance away. He was called "Uncle

---

30  Spina bifida (Latin: "split spine") is a developmental birth defect involving the neural tube: incomplete closure of the embryonic neural tube results in an incompletely formed spinal cord. <http://en.wikipedia.org/wiki/Spina_bifida> Accessed October 15, 2008.

31  2008. Dir. Sam Mendes. Plot summary: "A young couple living in a Connecticut suburb during the mid-1950s struggle to come to terms with their personal problems while trying to raise their two children. Based on a novel by Richard Yates." http://www.imdb.com/title/tt0959337/ Accessed October 22, 2009.

Warren" by Eli's parents. I have never been called "Aunt," and I doubt Eli knows I am his. I remember when an attendant called me "Aunt Romy" and Eli looked bewildered.

Once, Eli was eating grapes at a table. My mother asked if I could join him. He said no. I have had closer friendships with strangers' children than with my own nephew. A toddler in a stroller put a hand on the bar of my moving wheelchair in a mall. We immediately stopped moving. He gripped my handle bar, looked into my eyes, and smiled. My heart melted.

My mom commented later about Eli's wondering about a familial relationship, and I said I was not surprised. My dad asked me what I meant and I kept silent.

My mom once prepared what she labeled a "humanist" Passover Seder Dinner[32] (she even included an orange on the Seder Plate to symbolize the union of a lesbian couple joining us). All references to God were omitted lest they prove to be offensive to some members of my family. My mom has said that the Jewish holidays are about tradition—a link between the past and the future. The kids never celebrated Passover, Rosh Hashanah, Yom Kippur, or Hanukah with us again. We might have a dinner that excludes all allusion to a holiday. They came over for a pseudo-Rosh Hashanah dinner.[33] I felt badly for my mother because it had nothing to do with tradition. My parents and I have a traditional celebration on another night.

I adore the Jewish holidays. I personally think it is amazing to share in various cultures. I also think it is necessary to know

---

32 "The Passover Seder Meal (Hebrew: סֵדֶר, seðɛr, "order", "arrangement") is a Jewish ritual feast held on the first (and for some, the second) night of the Jewish holiday of Passover (which begins on the 15th day of Hebrew month of Nisan)." <http://en.wikipedia.org/wiki/Passover_Seder >Accessed Octobeer 22, 2009.

33 "Rosh Hashanah is the first of the High Holidays or *Yamim Noraim* ("Days of Awe"), or *Asseret Yemei Teshuva* (The Ten Days of Repentance) which are days specifically set aside to focus on repentance that conclude with the holiday of Yom Kippur." <http://en.wikipedia.org/wiki/Rosh_Hashanah> Accessed October 22, 2009.

one's heritage. Eli is half Jewish. Will he ever know that? It is not like anyone is trying to convert him or make him believe anything. It is odd to me because my brothers and I celebrated everything. I even went to a Hebrew school, yet we all are far from conventional. I often say that I am redefining the parameters for being Jewish. I was asked to be on a television show that explored Jewish life. To me, this was a great opportunity to show multiplicity in thought. *Anyway* … at least the children get to celebrate Christmas. Yup. My wish is that things will change for Tomek and that I will develop a relationship with Eli. Lately, after some time with me, Eli has warmed up. Hope is there.

If I were able-bodied, I would have a better relationship with my nephews. If I were able-bodied, I could run after the kids. I could play with them on their terms. It might take an effort on everybody's part to include me now. As I have said, life is not easy and I can only do so much. Socrates said, "Be as you wish to seem." To say that I am gravely disappointed in some relatives is an understatement.

# Chapter 16

## *Balancing Act*

THERE'S NO SECRET TO BALANCE.
YOU JUST HAVE TO FEEL THE WAVES.
—Frank Herbert

I WENT TO an osteopath. Lisa recommended him to me as her parents went to him, and we are both huge fans of osteopathy. "Osteopathy is an approach to healthcare that emphasizes the role of the musculoskeletal system in health and disease. In most countries osteopathy is a form of complementary medicine, emphasizing a holistic approach and the skilled use of a range of manual and physical treatment interventions (osteopathic manipulative medicine, or OMM in the United States) in the prevention and treatment of disease. In practice, this most commonly relates to musculoskeletal problems such as back and neck pain. Many osteopaths see their role as facilitating the body's own recuperative powers by treating musculoskeletal or somatic dysfunction."[34]

The osteopath said my torso was like a "Z" and my energy was flying to the left. He is aligning me. I felt a gravitas on my right side and a heaviness in the right side of my head I had never felt before. My hearing felt bizarre. My stomach gurgled, and

---

34  <http://en.wikipedia.org/wiki/Osteopathy>

my uterus tingled. The next day, I had increased energy. He is not suddenly going to make me walk—I do not expect that at all—but I like the connection. His work with my energy makes sense to me.

Even though the right side of my body is stronger and I favour it, I lean profoundly to the left when I eat or write. This is uncomfortable, painful, and limiting. Correcting this aspect is important and necessary. That someone is working on it is very meaningful to me.

Initially, as a creative visualization, he told me to inflate myself to the corners of the room, "like inflatable Romy." In this way, I imagined that my body was more receptive, more open to his work.

I am predisposed to certain qualities that pop up in osteopathy like creative visualization. Not only am I very familiar with it, but I like it a lot. I also really believe in the unseen energies of the body.

The next time I saw the osteopath, I fell asleep on the table for the first time in my life. I have a massage every week for circulation, and that does not happen to me. When an attendant came in later to help me off the table, she said that I looked different—like I had been on a journey and came back rejuvenated. She said my face was brighter, that I appeared energized. While I was having the treatment, many images came into my mind. It felt very physical, and that night I slept like a baby, as if I had run a marathon that day.

The osteopath did something to my leg and focused on my torso. My digestion was improved tremendously, and the most significant thing was that I reduced the amount of time I wore a night foot brace. I usually wore it five out of seven nights but reduced it to three out of seven nights. In *You Never Know*, I said,

I had foot surgery—to help me walk again—in June 2005. The doctor had to do a tendon transfer and an Achilles tendon lengthening. During the coma, my left foot went into a funny position with my toes pointed down. Called "dropped foot," it needed to be corrected. (Like I said, there are tons of surgical procedures now.) I tried to fix it in physiotherapy and with braces, but nothing worked. It still does not feel like the right foot, but it sure looks good. In addition to trying to negotiate the mixed-up signals to my brain with respect to balance and coordination, I have to negotiate this foot. It feels like it is turning, and there is some numbness on the bottom. Right now, a foot brace has been created for me that I wear all of the time. This brace prevents my foot from pointing down.[35]

I was referring to an old day-brace, but the night one is very similar.

The results only lasted one week because, as my physiotherapist says, my automatic body-regulator is flawed. I do believe osteopathy helps me occasionally but not like most people. The corrections to my body fluctuate as I do.

I really like to watch dance programs on the television, and I saw uber-gymnastic Cirque du Soleil's show *Ovo* in Old Montreal. I find feats of the body inspiring and hopeful. Watching people defy gravity and contort against seemingly impossible odds is rewarding to me. Because my own body is severely limited, I enjoy the examples of surpassing limitations and breaking through boundaries. I am the furthest from being a dancer or gymnast, yet merely the act of watching opens possibilities for me. An expectation might be that I would feel sad watching this stuff, but I do not.

Ovid said, "All things change, nothing is extinguished. There is nothing in the whole world which is permanent. Everything

---

35   *You Never Know: A Memoir*, p. 103.

flows onward; all things are brought into being with a changing nature; the ages themselves glide by in constant movement." Dancing reaffirms this to me.

When I was about fifteen, I studied modern dance at a place called the Dance Factory in Town of Mount Royal, on Lucerne Road. I had spent many youthful years studying ballet at the Eleanor *Ashton* School of *Dance,* so this felt freeing to me, but my classical training was a definite asset. When I studied musical theatre later on, I was really prepared for dance class. While I was capable, I was by no stretch of the imagination great. Now I will often say all of that training helps me.

# Chapter 17

## Worthy Estimation

I TRULY BELIEVE I have been underestimated intellectually my entire life. Because of my investment in image, fashion, camp, etc., I have been labeled as superficial or less than intelligent or deep. Someone I know from graduate school was apparently "surprised" by me when he read *You Never Know*. I still get comments from people who, I think, relegate me as "insipid." Someone compared me to Jane Austen's Emma. I am a big fan of Jane Austen, but the character of Emma lacks gravitas and is often mistaken in her own perceptions of the world around her. That is not me but is the perceived me. I am far from clueless.[36]

Some of my statistics are the following:

- I have a PhD from the University of Toronto. In addition, I have an MA from there. My BA is from McGill University.
- I am included in the *Bibliography of Theatre History in Canada.*

---

36 'Emma, Jane Austen's novel is modernized and given this very accurate title 'Clueless.'" <http://www.imdb.com/title/tt0112697/plotsummary> Accessed October 22, 2009.

- My article *"Drag King Invasion: Taking Back the Throne"* (CTR, Volume 86, Spring 1996, pp. 24–28) is in the book *Camp: Queer Aesthetics and the Performing Subject* (University of Michigan Press, 1999), which, as the promotional material states, "addresses the multilayered issue of camp, whose inexhaustible breadth of reference and theoretical relevance to the issues taken up by academic research in recent years..." In a very lucky way, my work has been appropriated by the gay community.
- I am in an issue (Fall '08) of *U of T Magazine*.
- My book *You Never Know: A Memoir* (Trafford, 2008) and story were featured on CBC News Sunday.
- I was reviewed as the feature artist for *You Never Know: A Memoir* in an issue of *Lipstik Indie*.
- As a pop culture critic, I wrote articles for magazines as diverse as *FAB* and *Canadian Theatre Review*.
- I am a contributor for Shebytches.com. I feel honoured on many levels for this. It is really important to diminish words that have been used to belittle, denigrate, humiliate, etc. The term *bitch* has been reappropriated and through this site is full of power and strength. (For example, many in the gay community have owned the word *queer*.) View current articles such as "Ogre-Drag," "POP Goes the Teen," "Double Standard?" "People Seem to Abhor 'Difference,'" and "Big Bother."
- I acted in a television series on YTV called *System Crash*.
- One of my articles has been translated into Italian and is used in the teaching of a university course on communications. A separate article is taught by Professor S. Scott at the University of Lethbridge in Alberta. It has also been chosen to be included in a book. I have been on the same course syllabus as Simone de Beauvoir.

A woman I know from high school believes her magnificent daughter is smarter than me. If I had looked very conservative things would have been different, I am sure. I was never a bookish student or a homely grad scholar. While studying drama for my master's and PhD, I was cast as a goddess in a theatrical production at school; this did not help matters. If I see a good-looking woman, I do not immediately think, "Oh, she must be smart." In fact, I think a prevalent belief is that she would be dumb. Even though I had confirmation, affirmation, and prejudice levied against me, I never felt beautiful. Someone I know from graduate school said she thought I was "drop-dead gorgeous." Sure.

According to the fabulous book *Third Wave Feminism and Television* by the head of women's studies at South Carolina University, Merri Lisa Johnson, I am a third-wave feminist. Who knew? I am quoted pretty extensively in there. I was researching what it meant to be a "third-wave feminist" and discovered that it involves an alignment with a survivor mentality rather than a victim mentality. By coincidence or not, I absolutely never felt like a victim.

Being called a third-wave feminist by an expert in a critical book was validating of my past, my life's work. It is only a part of my structure or process, but it has always been there. I won a book prize in high school and was given a book titled *Subject Woman* – a book of women's critical theory. I used to read a lot of women's critical theory. I was drawn to it from a very young age.[37] In the latter half of the 1990s, I wrote articles on gender-play and had a chapter on female camp in my doctoral dissertation.

I wrote the following before my doctoral dissertation. It was originally published in *Canadian Theatre Review* and the

---

37   Some of the above appears in my book *Again*, p. 63.

title was "A Drag King Invasion: Taking Back the Throne."[38] I performed female to female drag for research.

The terms *femme* and *butch* connote a "playing at" being female or male. Gender characteristics are heightened by the femme and the butch such that they foreground cultural gender prescriptions. Raising butch-femme role playing to the level of performative spectacle requires a leap from mere cross-dressing to drag, the elementary fabric of camp. Drag is not merely about dressing up as The Other, female dressing up as male and vice versa. Drag firmly plants one high heel or construction boot in ideology and one just outside of its grasp. Drag and camp performance embraces, and embraces and embraces the dominate culture's prescription for gender until it finally explodes and splatters itself all over the performer and spectator. Gender mess.

[C]amp is concerned with what might be called a philosophy of transformations and incongruity. (Newton, 105)[39]

I am very interested in the ways we can play at being female and male and found a book called *Pin-up Grrrls: Feminism, Sexuality, Popular Culture.* Its promotional material states, "Subverting stereotypical images of women, a new generation of feminist artists is remaking the pin-up, much as Annie Sprinkle, Cindy Sherman, and others did in the 1970s and 1980s. As shocking as contemporary feminist pin-ups are intended to be, perhaps more surprising is that the pin-up has been appropriated by women for their own empowerment since its inception more than a century ago."[40]

---

38   *Drag King invasion: taking back the throne,* CTR, Volume: 86, Pages: 24-28, illus.
39   *Drag King invasion: taking back the throne,* CTR, Volume: 86, Pages: 24-28, illus.
40   *Pin-up Grrrls: Feminism, Sexuality, Popular Culture,* by Maria Elena Buszek, May 2006, Duke University Press. <http://www.goodreads.com/book/show/452163.Pin_up_Grrrls_Feminism_Sexuality_Popular_Culture>

I remember a while ago I had a pin-up of Bettie Page on my fridge. She was very radical, so powerful. Much later, when a film came out about her, I saw it.[41]

It is very odd to be validated and lauded finally but completely dismissed and treated like a child as well. One of my attendants said that initially she was "shocked" by how young I appeared. Beforehand, she was told I was forty-three and expected a very different version of what that meant. She is a few years younger than me but says that I look at least twenty years younger than I am. Because I have a distorted vision of myself, I asked her if this affects some people's attitudes toward me. She acknowledged that if I appear younger, certain older people would feel terrible that this happened to a young person. Hmmm.

I was practicing walking with my physiotherapist in a carpeted hallway, and I took a short break on a seat. An elderly woman from an apartment nearby stopped to admire my earrings. She called me a "lucky little girl." Even if I looked twenty years younger, I would not be a little girl.

This infantilizing theme around me is so frustrating. Someone was pushing my wheelchair, and we saw a baby stroller. It was jokingly suggested that I should use one like it. Ha.

Okay, while I am discussing the "irritable"… people tend to think I should automatically bond with others in wheelchairs because of this commonality. Do all redheads or Canadians share the same perspective? I might share views with others in wheelchairs; I might not. The impulse here, as with infantilizing, comes from a good place, but it is ultimately demeaning.

41  *The Notorious Bettie Page* (Director: Mary Harron, 2005) Synopsis: "In an incandescent performance, Gretchen Mol (The Shape of Things) stars as Bettie Page, who grew up in a conservative religious family in Tennessee and became a photo model sensation in 1950s New York. Bettie's legendary pin-up photos made her the target of a Senate investigation into pornography, and transformed her into an erotic icon who continues to enthrall fans to this day." <http://www.newline.com/properties/thenotoriousbettepage.html > Accessed October 22, 2009.

I ran into someone at a movie theatre I had not seen in a long while. He had been told a few minutes earlier, by my father, what I had been through. He would not look at me. I am sure for him my situation was sad and shocking, but I ended up feeling ignored.

Even though I was no athlete, I went to the gym a lot for the sake of my physical appearance. Adjusting to this body is quite complex and often difficult because of the premium I used to place on my physicality. There are psychological components in addition to physical ones. Nevertheless, I see myself as an experiment in alternative lifestyles, and that is an indication of my belief system. Negotiating the physical is mental.

# Chapter 18

—•◆•—

## *Letting Go*

LETTING GO DOESN'T MEAN GIVING UP, BUT RATHER
ACCEPTING THAT THERE ARE THINGS THAT CANNOT BE.

—wolfdyke

I HAVE BEEN emotionally abandoned by many people in my life. My hardest lesson was understanding that for some friends to move on, they had to let go of me. As a direct result, I had to let go of them. Ouch. For me, this was a very painful process. Going against the grain, struggle, is not me. Acceptance, but not resting on my laurels, is. To let go with love in one's heart is a challenge. It has absolutely nothing to do with animosity or contention.

In the film *Titanic*,[42] Rose physically lets go of the dead Jack into the icy water while saying, "I'll never let go." We understand that a spiritual letting go is different from a physical letting go. My internal connection to these friends is solid and steadfast.

Part of me thinks I should be mean and get some "balls," but I cannot. Even though the pain is great, I cannot lash out. This goes for many things in my life. I heard a word applied to a situation, and although there might be a sense of bizarre comfort

---

42  1997, dir. James Cameron. Plot summary: "Fictional romantic tale of a rich girl and poor boy who meet on the ill-fated voyage of the 'unsinkable' ship." <http://www.imdb.com/title/tt0120338/> Accessed October 22, 2009.

in relegating everything to "dysfunction," I believe letting me go moves beyond that. Everything has its time. I might be able to adapt to change well, but not everyone is like that. Different circumstances necessitate different attitudes. Older structures do not apply in most cases. In many ways, I am the one who has gone forward; I had to alter to suit my current status. Even though older beliefs come into focus now, there are certain personalities that just do not fit well. Sure, it sucks. Yes, it is painful and hard—it is not pleasant. Life goes on, though.

### *It is odd to let go with love in your heart.*

I am beginning anew on so many levels. At the same time, I am not reinventing myself. It is like I am taking my older beliefs and adapting them to my new situation. As usual, I am in flux, and I do not mind changing my mind. I give myself permission to be flexible. People will often ask me if I believe such and such. I believe in exploration. When you explore, you might discover a new path you were not expecting.

I have had to let go a lot. Simply put, I have had to let go of the old me and much of what I did. Because they died, I will never see James, my eighteen-year-old cat Annie, or my grandparents ever again. I had a dream of having my own children. I will never give birth. I will never see my eight-year-old cat Leiloo again because she was given away during my coma. I know I will never sound as I did because of my dysarthria, so singing and speaking need to be revised. I will never sing opera again. My looks have altered—I have had to let go of my old image. I was physically attractive to people. I used to walk, run, jog, climb a Stairmaster, climb stairs, handwrite, write in a journal, write letters or postcards, type with both hands, have straight fingers, have a left foot that did not turn in, sign my entire name, swim in pools or lakes or the sea, dive, ski, snowboard, ice skate, roller skate, ballet dance, tap dance, jazz dance, club dance, do yoga, clap, snap my fingers, whistle, blow up a balloon, blow a kiss, blow a whistle, blow-dry my hair, hail a cab, drive a car, read without magnification, ride a bike, use a skateboard, pucker my lips, kiss, zip up a jacket, button a blouse, put on a coat, put on my own clothes, take a shower on my own, wash my own hair, brush my hair, use eyeliner and mascara, use dental floss, use Q-tips, read books and magazines and newspapers easily, read subtitles, see in a way that the world did not, bounce up and down, have a left eye that did not stay open all the time, not use eye drops constantly, have balance, drive a car, ride a bike, go camping, hike, portage, put up a tent, build a fire, throw a ball, catch a ball, stir soup, drink without a straw, cut my own food, use a knife, use scissors, use a stapler, use a telephone, use a cell phone, eat popcorn, suck on a mint or candy, chew gum, plant a vegetable garden, pick flowers, hum a tune … But I laugh a lot, and I find bliss in simple things. It can be very sad to let go. It is all in how you look at it.

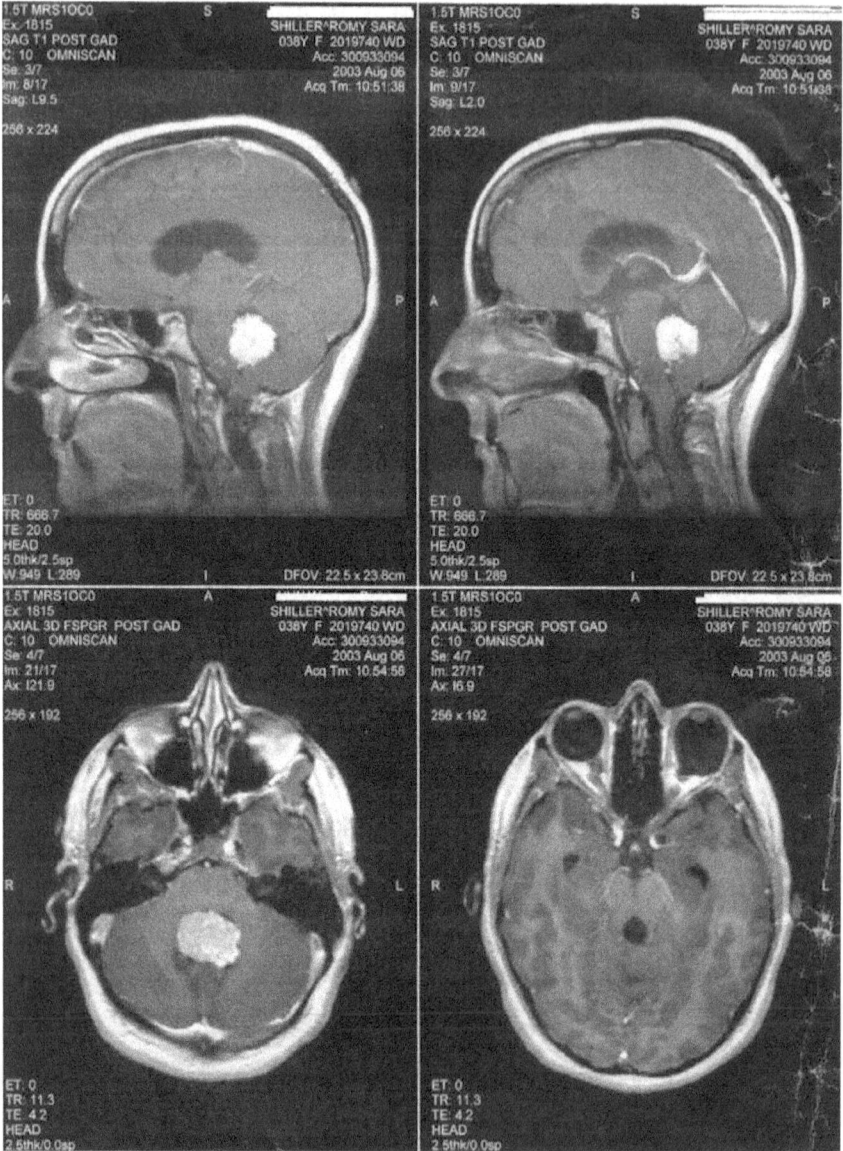

# Bibliography

## BOOKS

- **Buszek, Maria Elena.** 2006. *Pin-Up Grrrls: Feminism, Sexuality, Popular Culture.* Duke University Press.
- **Coupland, Douglas.** 1991. *Generation X: Tales for an Accelerated Culture.* St. Martin's Press.
- **Greene, Brian.** 1999. *The Elegant Universe: Superstrings, Hidden Dimensions, and the Quest for the Ultimate Theory.* Vintage.
- **Johnson, Merri Lisa.** 2007. *Third Wave Feminism and Television: Jane Puts It in a Box.* I. B. Tauris.
- **Lederman, Leon** and **Teresi, Dick.** 1993. *The God Particle: If the Universe Is the Answer, What Is the Question?* Dell Publishing.
- **Oakley, Ann.** *Subject Women.* Oxford: Martin Robertson, 1981.
- **Shiller, Romy.** 2009. *Again.* Trafford Publishing.
- ———. *Ooo La La.* Forthcoming.
- ———. 2008. *You Never Know: A Memoir.* Trafford Publishing.
- **Weiss, Brian L.** 1988. *Many Lives, Many Masters.* Simon and Schuster.
- **Weiss, Brian L.** 1993. *Through Time Into Healing.* Simon and Schuster.
- **Wilber, Ken.** 1984. *Quantum Questions: Mystical Writings of the World's Great Physicists..* Boston, MA: Shambhala Publications, Inc.

## DISSERTATION

**Shiller, Romy.** *A Critical Exploration of Cross-Dressing and Drag in Gender Performance and Camp in Contemporary North American Drama and Film.* National Library of Canada.

## MAGAZINES

**Boles, David W.** "Enforcing the Ugly Laws." <http://urbansemiotic.com/2007/05/01/enforcing-the-ugly-laws/> Accessed September 14, 2008.

**"Don't look now, but generation X is middle-aged."** Canada.com. *<http://www.canada.com/Entertainment/look+generation+middle+aged/2040937/story.html?id=2040937>* Accessed November 4, 2009.

**Damer, Bruce.** *"Avatars!* Exploring and Building Virtual Worlds on the Internet." Copyright Bruce Damer. 1998.

**"Maroon 5 frontman Adam Levine Discusses His Playboy Image, Onscreen Sex Scenes, Steamy New CD."** Dose.ca. <http://www.dose.ca/music/story.html?id=b97fd740-65e5-41db-9975-b576a24ab890> Accessed August 28, 2009.

**"Ashton and Demi: A Giant Step for Older Women?"** Ezine@articles. <http://ezinearticles.com/?Ashton-and-Demi:-A-Giant-Step-for-Older-Women?&id=85720> Accessed August 29, 2009.

**Herold, Edward S., Milhausen Robin R.** *Journal of Sex Research.* Nov, 1999.

**"Healthy Body Image: What Is Body Image?"** Peel Public Health. <http://www.peelregion.ca/health/commhlth/bodyimg/bintro.htm> Accessed August 31, 2009.

**Shiller, Romy.** "Double Standard?" July 27, 2009.

<http://www.shebytches.com/romyshillerjuly272009.html>

———. "Crush and Some Dualities." October 26, 2009. <http://www.shebytches.com/romyshilleroct262009.html>

———. "Drag King Invasion: Taking Back the Throne," *Canadian Theatre Review*, Spring 1996, Number 86, pp. 24–28.

———. "My 1980s." www.shebytches.com

———. "Ogre-Drag." April 26, 2009. <http://www.shebytches.com/romyshillerapr262009.html>

———. "POP Goes the Teen." June 29,2009. <http://www.shebytches.com/romyshillerjune2009.html>

———. "Why Is *Queer as Folk* Making Women Wet?" *FAB Magazine*, Number 213, April 23, 2003, pp. 12–17.

Schumaker, John F. 2008. "Star Struck." <http://findarticles.com/p/articles/mi_m0JQP/is_363/ai_111617817/> Accessed August 31, 2009.

The New York *Times.* "In Montreal, Where to Find What's Au Courant." <http://www.nytimes.com/1986/11/09/travel/shopper-s-world-in-montreal-where-to-find-what-s-au-courant.html> Accessed November 10, 2009.

## FILMS

Source: IMDb. http://www.imdb.com

*Aladdin.* Dirs. Ron Clements and John Musker. Walt Disney Feature Animation. 1992.

*Back to the Future.* Dir. Robert Zemeckis. Universal Pictures. 1985.

*Bernard and Doris.* Dir. Bob Balabanand. Trigger Street Independent. 2007.

*Bill & Ted's Excellent Adventure.* Dir. Stephen Herek. De Laurentiis Entertainment Group (DEG). 1989.

*Bridget Jones's Diary.* Dir. Sharon Maguire. Little Bird. 2001.

*Clueless.* Dir. Amy Heckerling. Paramount Pictures. 1995.

*Dirty Dancing.* Dir. Emile Ardolino. Great American Films Limited Partnership. 1987.

*Ghostbusters.* Dir. Ivan Reitman. Black Rhino Productions. 1984.

*Groundhog Day.* Dir. Harold Ramis. Columbia Pictures Corporation. 1993.

*Mammoth.* Dir. Tim Cox. Castel Film Romania. 2006.

*Minority Report.* Dir. Steven Spielberg. Twentieth Century-Fox Film Corporation. 2002.

*Nim's Island.* Dirs. Jennifer Flackett and Mark Levin. Walden Media. 2008.

*Perfume: The Story of a Murder.* Dir.Tom Tykwer. Constantin Film Produktion. 2006.

*Revolutionary Road.* Dir. Sam Mendes. BBC Films. 2008.

*Scaphandre et le papillon.* Dir. Julian Schnabel. Pathé Renn Productions. 2007.

*Sense and Sensibility.* Dir. Ang Lee. Columbia Pictures Corporation.1995.

*Sixteen Candles.* Dir. John Hughes. Channel Productions. 1984.

*Sliding Doors.* Dir. Peter Howitt. Intermedia Films. 1998.

*St. Elmo's Fire.* Dir. Joel Schumacher. Columbia Pictures Corporation. 1985.

*Titanic.* Dir. James Cameron. Twentieth Century-Fox Film Corporation. 1997.

*The Breakfast Club.* Dir. John Hughes. A&M Films. 1985.

*The Curious Case of Benjamin Button.* Dir. David Fincher. The Kennedy/Marshall Company. 2008.

*The Matrix.* Dirs. Andy Wachowski and Larry Wachowski. Groucho II Film Partnership. 1999.

*The Notorious Bettie Page.* Dir. Mary Harron. HBO Films. 2005.

*The Wizard of Oz.* Dir. Victor Fleming. Metro-Goldwyn-Mayer (MGM). 1939.

## TELEVISION

Source: IMDb. http://www.imdb.com

*The A-Team.* Creators: Stephen J. Cannell and Frank Lupo. Stephen J. Cannell Productions. 1983–1987.

*B.J. and the Bear.* Creators: Christopher Crowe and Glen A. Larson. Universal TV . 1979–1981.

*Cagney & Lacey.* Creators: Barbara Avedon and Barbara Corday. Columbia Broadcasting System (CBS). 1982–1988.

*Cheers.* Creators: James Burrows, Glen Charles, Les Charles, et al. Charles/Burrows/Charles Productions. 1982–1993.

*CHiPs.* Creator: Rick Rosner. MGM Television. 1977–1983.

*The Cosby Show.* Creators: Bill Cosby and Michael Leeson. Ed. Weinberger. Bill Cosby.1984–1992.

*Dallas.* Creator: David Jacobs. Lorimar Television. 1978–1991.

*Designing Women.* Writer: Bill Kenny (series). Bloodworth-Thomason. 1986–1993.

*Diff'rent Strokes.* Creators: Jeff Harris and Bernie Kukoff. Embassy Pictures Corporation. 1978–1986.

*Doogie Howser M.D.* Creators: Steven Bochco and David E. Kelley. Twentieth Century Fox Television. 1989–1993.

*The Facts of Life.* Creators: Dick Clair and Jenna McMahon. Embassy Pictures Corporation. 1979–1988.

*Family Ties.* Creator: Gary David Goldberg. Paramount Television.1982–1989.

*Fantasy Island.* Creator: Gene Levitt. Columbia Pictures Television. 1978–1984.

*Golden Girls.* Creator: Susan Harris. Touchstone Television. 1985–1992.

*Grey's Anatomy.* Creator: Shonda Rhimes. ABC. 2005–present.

*Hill Street Blues.* Creators: Steven Bochco and Michael Kozoll. MTM Enterprises. 1981–1987.

*House M.D.* Creator: David Shore. Heel & Toe Films. 2004–present.

*The Incredible Hulk.* Marvel Productions.1978–1982.

*Knots Landing.* Creator: David Jacobs. Columbia Broadcasting System (CBS).1979–1993.

*L.A. Law.* Creators: Steven Bochco and Terry Louise Fisher. Twentieth Century Fox Television. 1986–1994.

*Life on Mars.* Creators: Mathew Graham, Tony Jordan, and Ashley Pharoah. Kudos Film and Television. 2008–present.

*The Love Boat.* Writers: Buddy Akinson and Lee Aronsohn. Aaron Spelling Productions. 1977–1986.

*Married with Children.* Creators: Ron Leavitt and Michael G. Moye. Embassy Television. 1987–1997.

*Moonlighting.* Creator: Glenn Gordon Caron. ABC Circle Films. 1985–1989.

*Mork & Mindy.* Creators: Joe Glauberg, Garry Marshall, and Dale McRaven. Henderson Productions. 1978–1982.

*Prison Break.* Creator: Paul Scheuring. Rat Entertainment. 2005–2009.

*Quantum Leap.* Creator: Donald P. Bellisario. Belisarius Productions. 1989–1993.

*Queer as Folk.* Creators: Ron Cowen and Daniel Lipman. Cowlip Productions. 2000–2005.

*So You Think You Can Dance Canada.* Director: Nigel Lythgoe. SFA Productions. 2008–present.

*Star Trek: The Next Generation.* Creator: Gene Roddenberry. Paramount Television. 1987–1994.

*Three's Company.* Creators: Brian Cooke and Johnnie Mortimer. DLT Entertainment Ltd. 1977–1984.

*The Wonder Years.* Creators: Carol Black, Neal Marlens, et al. New World Television. 1988–1993.

## BLOGS

"Avatars for the wheelchair-bound: The value of inclusion in digital spaces." *Theory and Research in HCI.* http://comm6480rpi.blogspot.com/2008/10/avatars-for-wheelchair-bound-value-of.html> Accessed June 8, 2009.

"My 1980s – process." The Shebytches Articles. <http://rshiller.blogspot.com/> Accessed December 18, 2009.

"80's Pop Culture" http://onlythe80s.blogspot.com/ Accessed November 4, 2009.

## WEBSITES

http://books.google.ca/books?id=_4oKBQdqfBEC&dq=bust+magazine&source=gbs_summary_s&cad=0

http://eightiesclub.tripod.com/

http://en.wikipedia.org/wiki/Age_disparity_in_sexual_relationships

http://en.wikipedia.org/wiki/Aladdin_(film)

http://en.wikipedia.org/wiki/California_Proposition_8_(2008)

http://en.wikipedia.org/wiki/Coloratura

http://en.wikipedia.org/wiki/Doris_Duke

http://en.wikipedia.org/wiki/Jean-Dominique_Bauby

http://en.wikipedia.org/wiki/Grey%E2%80%99s_Anatomy

http://en.wikipedia.org/wiki/Le_Plateau-Mont-Royal

http://en.wikipedia.org/wiki/Maroon_5
http://en.wikipedia.org/wiki/Osteopathy
http://en.wikipedia.org/wiki/Passover_Seder
http://en.wikipedia.org/wiki/Rosh_Hashanah
http://en.wikipedia.org/wiki/Saint_Laurent_Boulevard
http://en.wikipedia.org/wiki/Spina_bifida
http://en.wikipedia.org/wiki/Sticky_&_Sweet_Tour
http://en.wikipedia.org/wiki/The_Holocaust
http://en.wikipedia.org/wiki/The_Notorious_Bettie_Page
http://en.wikipedia.org/wiki/Third_wave_feminism
http://en.wikipedia.org/wiki/Twitter
http://feminism.suite101.com/article.cfm/third_wave_feminism
http://findarticles.com/p/articles/mi_m2372/is_4_36/ai_58459537/
http://health.usnews.com/blogs/on-parenting/2009/05/26/
    girls-with-sexy-avatars-face-greater-risks-online.html
http://kidshealth.org/teen/food_fitness/problems/eat_disorder.html
http://thinkexist.com/quotations/beauty
http://thinkexist.com/quotations/body/
http://thinkexist.com/quotes/with/keyword/image/
http://thinkexist.com/quotes/ingrid_bergman/2.html
http://thinkexist.com/quotations/friendship/
http://thinkexist.com/quotes/with/keyword/movement/
http://thinkexist.com/quotes/with/keyword/picture/
http://thinkexist.com/quotes/with/keyword/singing/2.htm
http://urbansemiotic.com/2007/05/01/enforcing-the-ugly-laws/
http://www.aardvarkarchie.com/quotes/sex.htm
http://www.adherents.com/people/pm/Madonna.html
http://www.advocate.com/article.aspx?id=36899
http://www.allsubs.org/search-movie-quotes/Suspended%20
    Animation%20/
http://www.associatedcontent.com/article/1048385/
    celebrities_fight_to_protect_gay_marriage.html?cat=2

http://www.bewebaware.ca/english/OnlinePredators.aspx#a2\
http//www.brainyquote.com/quotes/keywords/singer.html
http://www.brainyquote.com/quotes/quotes/w/
   wentworthm294279.html
http://www.bratz.com/
http://www.cbc.ca/sunday/2008/05/051108_3.html
http://www.famousquotes.me.uk/macbeth/14-macbeth-quote-
   look-like-the-innocent-flower.htm
http://www.goodreads.com/book/show/452163.Pin_up_
   Grrrls_Feminism_Sexuality_Popular_Culture
http://www.goodreads.com/quotes/show/66493
http://www.imdb.com/
http://www.imdb.com/title/tt0087332/quotes
http://www.imdb.com/title/tt0107048
http://www.imdb.com/title/tt0114388/
http://www.imdb.com/title/tt0120148/plotsummary
http://www.imdb.com/title/tt0120338/
http://www.imdb.com/title/tt0181689/
http://www.imdb.com/title/tt0401383/
http://www.imdb.com/title/tt0410377
http://www.imdb.com/title/tt0412142/
http://www.imdb.com/title/tt0421715/
http://www.imdb.com/title/tt0455275
http://www.imdb.com/title/tt0787490/
http://www.imdb.com/title/tt0959337/
http://www.imdb.com/title/tt1023481/fullcredits#cast
http://www.ix625.com/matrixscript.html
http://www.liketotally80s.com/
http://www.makefive.com/categories/entertainment/television/
   best-80s-tv-shows
http://www.newline.com/properties/thenotoriousbettepage.html

http://www.nytimes.com/1986/11/09/travel/shopper-s-world-in-montreal-where-to-find-what-s-au-courant.html

http://www.popsugar.com/1634193

http://www.quotegarden.com/age.html

http://www.quotegarden.com/conformity.html

http://www.quotegarden.com/food.html

http://www.slate.com/id/2111753

http://www.squidoo.com/1980s-movie-quotes

http://www.thesite.org/sexandrelationships/havingsex/sexanddisability/sexwhenyouredisabled

http://www.worldofquotes.com/topic/infatuation/index.html

http://www.worldofquotes.com/topic/materialism/index.html

www.ingramcontent.com/pod-product-compliance
Lightning Source LLC
Chambersburg PA
CBHW071136280326
41935CB00010B/1248